The Sound of Silence

The Sound of Silence

journeys through miscarriage

Edited by Irma Gold

The Sound of Silence: Journeys Through Miscarriage
Published by Mostly for Mothers,
a division of Wombat Books
P. O. Box 1519, Capalaba Qld 4157
www.mostlyformothers.com
www.wombatbooks.com.au

First published 2011
Copyright belongs to individual authors
Edited by Irma Gold
Design and layout by Wombat Books

Ebook edition ISBN: 978-1-921632-12-9

National Library of Australia Cataloguing-in-Publication entry
Title: The sound of silence : journeys through miscarriage / editor, Irma Gold.
ISBN: 9781921632112 (pbk.)
Subjects: Miscarriage--Anecdotes.
Other Authors/Contributors: Gold, Irma.
Dewey Number: 362.198392

All rights reserved. No part of this publication may be reproduced, stored in, or introduced into a retrieval system, or transmitted, in any form, or by any means (electronic, mechanical, photocopying, recording or otherwise) without the prior written permission of the publisher.

An earlier version of 'Black Holes—The Art of Losing Babies' first appeared in *Meanjin.*

*For Rafael,
and all the other babies we have never met
but will always remember*

Contents

Introduction	vii
Falling	
Enza Gandolfo	1
False Starts	
Rebecca Freeborn	17
The Worry Space	
Gillian Freeman	28
Dissolve	
Melinda Small	34
What Starts with 'L' and Ends in Chemotherapy?	
Sarah Hart	37
A Blanket of Words	
Heidi Silberman	46

Black Holes—The Art of Losing Babies
Anne Myers 52

Not Talia
Melissa Ferguson 61

If the Blood had Come
Karen Andrews 69

The Detour
Christine Darcas 73

This Path Before
Tiffany Tregenza 85

For Tristan: A Meditation on Loss, Grief and Healing
Nicole Breit 90

On Reflection
Christine O'Neil 97

Letting Go
Choe Brereton 103

The Visitor
Sally O'Brien 107

Swords, Guns and Superheros
Becki Brown 114

A Perfect Square
Rosalind McKenzie 121

Sorrow Comes Unsent For
   Lou Pollard   124

Butterfly Nets
   Tracey Slater   128

Escaping from Good Friday
   Heather Murray Tobias   135

Unexpected
   Clare McHugh   143

The Long Wait
   Deb Nurton   152

Information and resources   159

Introduction

I am lying in a hospital bed, miscarrying. In the bed next to me lies another woman, also miscarrying. The curtain between us offering the pretence of privacy renders her faceless, but I cannot help overhear her conversations. It is her first pregnancy and, as she speaks to the doctor, behind her words I hear the vivid tapestry of her unspoken fears.

When the doctor leaves she cries, spills versions of these fears onto her partner. She is worried that there is something wrong with her, that the miscarriage is somehow her fault. I want to reach over, pull the curtain back, and comfort her. I already have two healthy children, and I know the statistics. Miscarriage is common. One in three pregnancies will end in miscarriage[1]. I *am* that statistic. And yet it's not that simple, losing a baby never is.

---
1   Statistics vary between one in five to one in two pregnancies. However one in three or four is more commonly cited.

In Australia alone women have about 55,000 miscarriages each year, yet the subject is taboo, both at a personal and public level. Women often keep their pregnancy a secret for the first twelve weeks in case something 'goes wrong'. The unfortunate consequence is that they must then grieve alone, silently, unable to talk about a baby they never openly declared. And because miscarriage is such a 'secretive' business, there is a lack of information, support and understanding available. So this private grief gets gagged, buried, overlooked, dismissed, stuffed into small corners—only to bubble up at unexpected moments.

Even if you do try to talk openly about your loss no one wants to hear. As I quickly discovered after losing my baby, people don't know what to say, or how to be with you. It makes them uncomfortable. It makes them nervous.

The result is often well-meant but unhelpful platitudes. The phrase 'Don't worry, you'll have another baby' is commonly offered up by nurses, doctors, friends and family in an attempt to help. It doesn't. One baby doesn't replace another. They are not objects. It's not like replacing a broken glass or a toy that no longer works. When you've carried a human being inside you, the grief does not evaporate with the arrival of a new baby, as many women within these pages can attest. The fact that we expect it to, that people so often readily dismiss miscarriage, denies women their right to grieve, and to acknowledge—in that moment, and in years to come—the child they lost.

'It's all for the best,' they also say (a phrase you'll find running through this anthology like an echo). The child that has been lost was not fit for this world, was defective, was just a bundle of malformed cells. So it's *all for the best*. In medical terms this may be true, but having rocked a baby inside your womb, it cannot be explained away with these words. It was a part of you, and its loss was real.

Shortly after I miscarried I explained what had happened to a friend in her sixties. She leaned closer to me, lowered her voice, and in hushed tones confessed the secret of her own miscarriage many decades before. We were the only two people in the room. This, to me, said it all. Miscarriage is an unspeakable subject.

So here we are. Speaking about it.

The Sound of Silence focuses on early pregnancy loss. There is the tendency to group together all kinds of infant loss—miscarriage, stillbirth and neonatal death—but this means that women who have experienced a miscarriage often feel that their loss is not as valid, that others have experienced far worse. And yet the grief remains.

After calling for submissions to this anthology women's stories flooded in. The need to speak was undeniable. The range of experiences shown here demonstrates that every miscarriage is unique, and yet the need to acknowledge those babies, and be allowed to grieve them openly, is the same. I thank all those who so bravely put pen to paper. It was a privilege to read your stories.

And I have no doubt that the twenty-two stories included here will move you. Within them you will not only find sorrow. You will also find hope and joy, strength and courage, and, most of all, overwhelming love.

In a way this anthology is my attempt to comfort that unknown woman I shared a hospital room with. I will never know if she reads this, but I hope that those of you who do find what you need. Together, we honour all those babies we have lost, and all those women who carried them.

Irma Gold
Editor

Falling

Enza Gandolfo

I grew up believing that if you put your mind to it, you can do anything.
 Setting goals.
 Working hard.
 Not giving up.

It's the miscarriage, not the pregnancy, which resembles a fall.
 I'm walking along the street admiring the neighbours' gardens, taking note of the new café on the corner, and then I trip. Unable to regain myself, I fall. I get up, there doesn't seem to be much damage. No one notices, and I keep going as if nothing happened. It's only the next day when I wake up that I feel the pain.

Some days I tell people I never expected having a baby would be so difficult.

Some days I tell people I always suspected I was infertile. In all those earlier more promiscuous years, while friends battled with decisions over unplanned pregnancies, I never got pregnant, even though I wasn't always careful.

I am in my mid-thirties when we start trying to get pregnant.

It takes over a year.

I don't know I am pregnant until after I miscarry.

Driving across town to meet friends for dinner, the cramps are so bad I have to turn around and go home.

The next day the doctor says, *You had a spontaneous abortion, a miscarriage.*

The blood test confirms it.

It's not unusual, she says. *Many women miscarry without even realising. They just shrug it off as a bad period. At least you know you can get pregnant.*

Her silver lining on my cloud.

I tell myself it will be fine.

Not a problem. Just a glitch.

Like a rain shower in the summer.

No worries, the doctor says. *Go forth and multiply.*

The day after the first miscarriage we are having a joint garage sale with close friends. For weeks we've been walking through the house looking for things we no longer need, things we can do without. In the morning we drag all our unwanted belongings across the neighbourhood: a suitcase full of clothes, several boxes of books, a dressmaker's dummy I bought in my twenties when I thought I might sew for a living, a side table we picked up at Camberwell market, a silver-plated cutlery set we were given for a wedding present, odd glasses, half-empty tins of paint. Our things join theirs—bits of discarded furniture, crockery, glasses, toys their kids have outgrown—until their driveway is a trash and treasure market. Buyers come early and bargain hard.

I feel tired and emotional. On the edge of tears.

It's the hormones, my friend says.

Full breasts. Tiredness.

And an overwhelming desire to go to bed, to hide under the blankets, to cry.

I go home before morning tea. I can't keep it together. I don't make it to my friend's birthday party that afternoon. Instead I spend most of the day sobbing.

Relentless tears. A flood.

The grief is more shocking than the miscarriage itself.

It takes almost another year for me to get pregnant again.

I love the texture of my pregnant skin.

I'm excited. Joy rises unexpectedly.

I smile, grin, laugh.

I feel giddy with the pleasure of it.

I try not to worry.

    I worry all the time.

    Some days I am too scared to move.

I think it's a girl.

    I think she should be named after our mothers, Domenica Rosa.

    I call her Nici for short.

    I talk to her. Long fleshy conversations.

As soon as the test is positive my GP sends me to a gynaecologist. It is a Monday morning when I arrive for my first appointment. There are two other women—both noticeably pregnant—in the waiting room. Their bellies are round and firm, their clothing stretches to the limit. There are a couple of toddlers playing, they have emptied the contents of the toy box onto the floor—there are dolls and stuffed toys, trucks and cars, giant blocks and thick cardboard picture books.

    The gynaecologist is a woman—I insisted—in her forties. In her straight blue skirt and white shirt, she looks like a bank teller. She introduces herself to me as we make our way into her office.

    Congratulations, she says. I smile. Grin.

    Until she suggests an ultrasound.

    One miscarriage is quite common, she says. *Doesn't mean you'll have any more problems but I think we should see how you're going.*

For the ultrasound I have to walk several blocks down the street from the clinic. The street—with the hospital on one side—is lined on the other side with weatherboard and brick veneer houses converted into offices for medical staff. Here I can have blood taken, I can have x-rays and ultrasounds, I can visit oncologists, cardiologists and immunologists.

The receptionist gives me a jug with two litres of water.

Drink it all, she says.

I drink and wait. And then when the drinking becomes too much I walk and drink and wait. My bladder is full. I walk in circles around the waiting room. I walk out into the back car park. I walk along the fence line. I talk to myself. I stroke my belly. I talk to Nici.

Hey kiddo, hang in there.

I tell myself not worry. That women have babies every day.

That everything is fine.

That Nici is going to be okay.

The technician moves the ultrasound across my stomach and abdomen. My eyes are on the screen. My focus is on my bladder which feels as if it is about to burst. I think about begging to be allowed to go to the toilet.

On the screen, the landscape of my womb is black and white, there are lines and hollows, there are waves. He takes measurements, he zooms in and out, his expression gives nothing away.

How many weeks do you think you are?

Seven, maybe eight. Is anything wrong?

I'll send the report over to the doctor, he says. *Best if you talk to her.*

He doesn't tell me Nici is fine.

I race to the toilet and then to the clinic. The toys are still scattered across the floor but the waiting room is now empty. I watch the doctor as she watches the report come out of the fax machine, as she reads it. I watch her slip the paper into my file.

Come in, she says and waits until we are both seated.

The foetus stopped growing—a few weeks ago.

I already knew this was what she was going to say. I already knew but I wanted to stop her saying the words. I wanted to gag her.

A spontaneous abortion, probably at six weeks.

Spontaneous, spontaneity.

Occasionally I do something on a whim, without planning, but only small inconsequential things.

I want to tell her that I do not have a particularly spontaneous nature.

I want to tell her it's taken me and my husband almost ten years to decide to have a baby.

That it took another year to get pregnant.

I want to tell her that for two weeks at least I have been talking to a dead foetus.

But I don't say anything.

If I speak I will cry and I don't want to cry in front of the doctor.

It's not unusual. It's much better to miscarry at this early stage. A miscarriage happens because something is wrong with the foetus. It's not unusual for women to have a couple of miscarriages.

I stop listening. I can see she is talking. I can see she is moving her mouth but I don't know what she is saying. I look over her head at the photographs of babies on the pin board behind her desk.

Tiny babies, carried by smiling mothers.

But there is no photograph of Nici.

No grainy ultrasound print to take home, to put on the fridge, to show my parents, my friends.

The receptionist makes an appointment for a curette at the end of the week.

At home I tell my husband, *I have lost the baby*.

Lost the baby.

Lost.

I lost my grandmother's watch.

I lost my mother's antique brooch.

I'm always losing my keys. Some mornings, already late for work, I turn the house upside down looking for them. My room looks like thieves have been on a rampage.

I lose time daydreaming.

I lose sleep worrying about all the things that might happen, could happen.

I'm often getting lost, even in my own city.

Did I lift something heavy? Swim too long? Work too many hours, was I too stressed?

How did I lose Nici?

I crawl into bed and cry.

The day the curette is scheduled, my husband takes the day off work.

We are one of three couples. We wait together to have the remains of our pregnancies scraped away.

Nothing to worry about, the doctor says when she passes me on the trolley as I wake up. *Just keep trying.*

It's only a miscarriage, I tell myself.

I list other people's losses.

I tell myself I have a good life.

I tell myself I am one of the lucky ones.

I give myself a good talking to.

Trying to have a baby takes over my life.

Each month.

Plot the cycle.

Sex by the calendar.

Waiting.

Every month there are the premenstrual cramps and blood, and a growing sorrow.

Women I've known all my life tell me stories I've never heard.

There are miscarriages everywhere.

One in three pregnancies, the gynaecologist says.

But all these stories seem to end in babies.
Babies.
There are babies everywhere.
Everyone seems to have a baby.

In the next waiting room there are no toys.
Here unpregnant couples sit in silence.
There are none of the breastfeeding, rubella injection, quit smoking half-torn posters that cover the walls of my gynaecologist's western suburbs waiting room.
But she's thrown her hands up in the air and referred me on.
This doctor is a fertility specialist. A man. In his thirties. His office is in the city.
He is one of the best, she tells me.

He does blood tests.
Finds a problem.
Gives it a name.
Antiphospholipid antibody syndrome.
He sits behind a wide empty desk.
He pulls a notepad out of the draw, a pen from his pocket. And he makes notes.
Antiphospholipid antibody syndrome?
It's a clotting disorder. When the body recognises a foreign substance it creates antibodies to neutralise it. Blood clots form in the placenta and starve the foetus.
Can you do anything about it?

My womb is a traitor.
> While I long for a baby, my womb is starving her.
> I am starving my baby.
> Bad mother.
> Baby killer.

Women with this condition go on to have children, the doctor says without looking up from his notebook.
> I wonder what he is writing.
> Maybe he is a poet.
> A magician.
> Maybe he can conjure up our baby with his words.

There are new rituals now.
> Ovary stimulating pills.
> Urine and blood tests.
> Weekly visits to a small cubicle in the city.
> Where I put my legs up in stirrups.
> And the doctor sits in a chair between my legs.
> He inserts the ultrasound probe and my womb fills the screen.
> The doctor is on a quest, for ovarian follicles, for ovulation.
> I have sex according to his instructions.

When finally I fall pregnant he says, *We've got you pregnant.*
> We.
> *We need to start the Heparin. It's the only hope.*
> Self-injecting twice a day.

I practice injecting an orange.
You'll be fine, the nurse says.

Heparin causes bruising.
The needle pierces my skin, and disappears.
Twice a day, twelve hours apart, morning and night.
My husband prepares the syringe.
I do the injecting.
Awkward, tedious procedure.
We have to be home at seven each morning, at seven each night.
Syringe, heparin, ice cubes.

Heparin to the rescue.
With each injection, I imagine Nici becoming stronger, growing.

A sentry of tiny purple blotches.
An ultrasound.
And finally—
A heartbeat.
Yes!

Every moment there is joy and fear.
Worry and wishing.
Some days I can't get out of bed.
I spend a week holding my breath.

But then ...

Blood. Dripping.
Dark red.
Falling.

My husband is asleep in the bed next to me. I don't know whether to wake him or not.

Is this an emergency? Should I ring triple zero? Should I call an ambulance? Should I rush to the hospital?

There are no cramps.

There is no pain.

My breasts are still tender and full.

I hear the wind and the rain.

I hear a dog barking.

I hear the swish of the fruit bat's wings as it flies across our driveway on its nightly journey between two peach trees.

I go to the bathroom and check again and again. Hoping the spotting is part of a nightmare.

But there it is.

Red. Blood.

Nici. Nici.

Nici.

I lie flat on the bed. My hand on my belly and I call her name.

Again and again.

I talk to my daughter.

I tell her stories, past and future. I tell her about her

grandmothers, Sicilian and Calabrese, two southern Italian women who came to Australia for a new life. For her new life.

We arrive at the clinic as the receptionist unlocks the door. My husband explains and we jump the queue.

I'm bleeding, I tell the doctor while we are still standing. *Just a few spots.*

I'll send you for an ultrasound, he says, sitting down to write a referral. *Find out what's going on. Come straight back with the results.*

I'd hoped for some words of reassurance, of comfort. He is not that sort of doctor, not that sort of man.

The waiting room is full.

There are several very pregnant women and their male partners.

There are toddlers and babies.

There is so much noise.

This time they don't make me drink any water at all.

They don't make me wait my turn.

How many weeks pregnant do you think you are? the technician asks.

I hate the way they ask that question—*do you think?*

Am I deluded? Has my body fooled me again?

Nine.

The technician's focus is on the computer screen.

I grip the side of the bed.

The sac is small. There's no heartbeat. I'm sorry.

The technician leaves the room.

My husband puts his arm around my shoulder.

Please don't say anything. Let's get out of here.

While I dress, neither of us speaks. What can we say?

I am afraid to speak.

The only way I can keep myself together is to say nothing.

To focus on breathing. To focus on making it out of the building.

The technician returns and shows us into a small empty room.

Wait here and I'll organise the report for the doctor.

We can hear the waiting room noise through the wall.

I guess this is the bad news room.

Outside someone cries out, *Twins, oh my God.*

This is followed by laughter and clapping.

We should try IVF, the doctor says.

How will that help?

It's taking too long for you to get pregnant, you'll run out of time. One of my patients with your condition had eight miscarriages before she had a baby.

Eight? I say.

If you really want to have a baby, you'll need to do IVF. And then the heparin as soon the embryo is implanted.

IVF doesn't always work.

Women who get pregnant on IVF would never get pregnant without it.

We are talking in circles.

I feel myself slipping.

Eight miscarriages. I can't imagine what kind of strength that would take. I don't think I have it.

We leave the doctor's room without making any decisions.

Later we discover that a side effect of heparin is osteoporosis. That some women who have been on it have bone fractures while sitting still.

If you really want to have a baby.

Really.

You'll do anything.

Give anything.

Take anything.

Set goals.

Work hard.

Believe in yourself.

It's a mantra and you see it everywhere.

But now I begin to think maybe …

Maybe it takes more courage to know when to stop.

To stop.

To accept that you can't control everything.

That not getting what you want is not the worst thing that can happen to you.

That life is chance.

That there is no *miscarriage* of justice here.

But some days I can still see Nici.

Even if she was only ever a figment of my imagination.

And never a real baby.

Some days I feel myself falling ...

Enza Gandolfo is a Senior Lecturer in Creative Writing at Victoria University, Melbourne. Her debut novel, Swimming *(Vanark Press, 2009), was shortlisted for the Barbara Jefferis Award in 2010. Her previous books include:* Inventory: On Op Shops *with Sue Dodd (Vulgar Press, 2007) and* It Keeps Me Sane: Women Craft Wellbeing *with Marty Grace (Vulgar Press, 2009). Her short stories, essays, autobiographical pieces, reviews and articles have been published in a range of literary journals, magazines and newspapers. Visit her at www.enzagandolfo.com*

False Starts

Rebecca Freeborn

I never expected to fall pregnant so quickly.

It took us eleven years to make the enormous, life-changing decision to have children. We got married and decided that as soon as we got back from our honeymoon, we'd start trying. I'd had a contraceptive implant and no periods for six years, so we both assumed it would take a while. Six months, maybe longer.

It took two weeks.

It wasn't quite the emotional, teary scene I'd imagined when I saw that first positive pregnancy test. For one thing, the line on the test was so faint we had to tilt it and hold it up to the light just to see it. A line is a line, said the instructions in the box. And the articles on the internet. And the people on the pregnancy forums. So I guess I was pregnant.

But I think it's safe to say neither of us was prepared for it.

'Bloody hell,' George said. About seven or eight times.

As for me, I was in a state of disbelief. Sure, my body had been doing all sorts of weird things over the last few weeks, so I knew *something* was up. But I couldn't reconcile those twinges—the waves of exhaustion, my sudden superpower sense of smell—with an actual infant. It all seemed so *unlikely*.

Nevertheless, I did all the things first-time expectant mothers do. I calculated my due date (going by the date of my last period, I was approximately six years and two weeks pregnant). I worked out when I'd be able to finish up at work. I tried to imagine how we'd transform the spare room from a CD and wine repository into a baby's room. I leapt ahead mentally by nine months. It simply never occurred to me that something might go wrong.

We were going interstate to visit friends several days after we found out, so I hadn't made an appointment with my GP yet. I'd done another pregnancy test, and the line was darker than last time, so I figured everything was fine and the appointment could wait until we got back.

I was at work on the day we were to leave when I discovered every pregnant woman's worst nightmare: I was bleeding.

Cue spiralling panic, sickening dread.

I was due to get on a plane in three hours. There wasn't even time to get to a doctor. And so I spent the next few hours googling madly, trying to find some evidence that would allay my fears. But the results brought me little comfort. Yes, bleeding in early pregnancy is common, but it's also one of the first and most common signs of miscarriage.

By the time we got to the airport, the bleeding had stopped. I allowed myself to think that everything was fine. And indeed, I spent the next few days in Melbourne feeling tired and queasy. That seemed like a good sign.

On the final day, I started to feel achy and had a sore throat. By the time we got home every part of my body was screaming with pain, particularly my lower back. It was like a bad period times a million. Finally, when I couldn't stand it any longer, I sent George out to the chemist to get some paracetamol.

'While you're there, could you get another pregnancy test?' I asked him before he left. I wanted to make absolutely sure before I went to the doctor.

The painkillers worked enough to get me to sleep and, other than the sore throat, I felt almost normal again in the morning. Until I did that pregnancy test. The line had retreated, become barely visible.

'I think I might be having a miscarriage,' I said to George when I went back to bed.

He just hugged me. I don't think he knew what to say. I didn't know what to say.

I couldn't get in to see my GP for another three days, so in the meantime I took pregnancy tests compulsively every morning. They kept getting fainter. One morning I realised I no longer had any pregnancy symptoms. By the time I went for my appointment, I'd pretty much reconciled myself to the fact that I'd lost the baby.

My doctor did a blood test, and she spoke about remaining hopeful. I could still be pregnant. A line is a line, after all. But I could tell, beneath her compassionate exterior, that she didn't think it was likely.

Nevertheless, I couldn't help nurturing a tiny spark of hope while I waited for the results. The doctor called me the following morning. She spoke in a low voice, and that's when I knew.

'Your HCG level is only four, which is far too low to be a viable pregnancy,' she said. 'I'm very sorry, but you'll probably experience a miscarriage in the next week.'

I was surprised by how well I took this news. It wasn't entirely unexpected, but I didn't feel the searing sense of loss I'd anticipated. I met George for lunch and calmly broke the news to him, even making a crack that at least now I could have a glass of wine.

It didn't really hit me until the following night. My period had come that morning, leaving me feeling as if I'd never been pregnant at all. As if I'd just imagined the whole thing. George stayed out late at work drinks and came home tipsy and in fine spirits. His mood was like a physical blow after what had happened. Sure, I hadn't exactly let him know how I was feeling—I didn't really know myself—but how could he move on like this, as if nothing had happened? Was part of him relieved that the complication had been removed?

He misinterpreted my surliness for annoyance at him being out late, and proceeded to lecture me about tolerating the demands of his work. It was all networking, he was doing it for us, et cetera. But his words seemed meaningless, unimportant. I started crying, and once I'd started I couldn't stop. Finally, George realised what was really going on.

'I feel it too,' he said.

Over the next few weeks, I sank into a deep depression. I told my best friend, Rachacia, what had happened, but other than that I kept everything inside and tried to act normally. But suddenly it seemed that every second woman on the street was pregnant, or had a baby. Each of them was an individual punch in the guts, a reminder of what I hadn't been able to do.

Then, to top it all off, Rachacia announced that she was pregnant. I tried to be gracious about it. And I was happy for her, really I was. But I couldn't help all the bad feelings from crowding in. Jealousy, resentment. Shame at my own reaction. Terror that something would go wrong with her pregnancy and I'd feel somehow responsible.

I finally told my other close friends about the miscarriage, and talking about it did help me to feel more positive, less alone. I figured the best way to get over it was to get pregnant again as soon as possible.

My cycle was all messed up, so I had no idea when I was ovulating, or when I could expect my period. Nevertheless, around six weeks after the miscarriage, I found myself with yet another positive pregnancy test. Again, the line was very faint, but this time I was more confident. This time, everything was going to go according to plan.

I noticed that George was a little reserved. He didn't speak much about the pregnancy, and warned me not to get my hopes up too high, just in case. But I couldn't help it. I'd read all the articles. I knew the chances of having a second miscarriage weren't any higher than the chance of having one. It'd be different this time. It was meant to be.

We shared the news with Rachacia and her partner. I was feeling good. We'd be pregnant together, just as we'd hoped, and have our babies only six weeks apart. No one could have planned it better.

During the week, my throat started to hurt as if I was getting a cold, but it never progressed into anything. I couldn't help feeling a cold prickle of foreboding. The last time I'd had a sore throat, I'd had a miscarriage a few days later. I pushed the thought away. It was just a coincidence. There was no way the two could be related.

That weekend, I was driving towards home when I had to pull over to use a public toilet. I was still at the stage where constant peeing was a cause for smug satisfaction rather than irritation. *You're so pregnant, girlfriend*, I congratulated myself as I walked in. But my triumph was short-lived—to my horror the toilet paper came away bright red. I was bleeding again.

I was barely aware of the rest of the drive, but somehow I found myself at home, and the situation couldn't have been worse. George had been having a boys' afternoon at our place, and I returned to a backyard full of loud, drunk blokes. I managed to get a moment alone with George and told him what had happened.

'I'm sure it's nothing,' he said with the kind of bravado that only doubt can fuel. 'If you think about it, it'd be weird if you didn't have *some* bleeding.'

In a way, his words made sense. I'd read countless stories online of women who'd bled during their pregnancies and still had healthy babies. But I just knew it wasn't the case for me.

I could feel it happening all over again.

The bleeding hadn't stopped by the next morning, and George insisted I go to a doctor. I didn't have the heart to tell him there was no point, that nothing could save the pregnancy now. We managed to find a surgery that was open on a Sunday, and saw a doctor who seemed more interested in pumping through as many patients as possible than actually doing anything to help. I don't think he even believed I was pregnant—he seemed convinced I was just having a late period and the pregnancy test was wrong. He told me to rest for the next two days and we were dismissed. I walked out feeling more upset than when we'd arrived.

That day was one of the worst of my life. It was as if all the grief I'd stored away from the last time had combined with this miscarriage to create a gaping, aching hole. I felt as if my heart had been wrenched out, put back in and allowed to heal, only to be ripped out all over again. I cried in the shower until my head throbbed. I couldn't speak or communicate with George, no matter how many times he tried. It was a hard-edged, raw anguish that ate at me from the inside out.

The following morning I used my last pregnancy test to confirm what I already knew—there was no longer a pregnancy. George and I lay side-by-side on the bed, neither of us knowing how to comfort the other except by being there.

'I don't know how I'm going to get through this again,' I said to him.

He asked me if I wanted him to stay at home with me, but I couldn't face another day with nothing but that to focus on. So, as foolish as it was, I went straight back to work. The only way I could keep my mind off what had happened was to throw myself into work and push everything else aside. And it did help, somewhat.

Rachacia sent me a text message during the week. *How's the little poppy seed going?* she asked. *No good*, I replied. *Another one bites the dust.*

I wallowed in self-pity for a long time, far longer than I should have. I withdrew from Rachacia, unable to bear hearing the details of her own pregnancy. I knew I was being unfair—she had a right to share her happiness, and I should have understood that—but her normal, healthy pregnancy was like a reproach to me. My behaviour drove a wedge into our friendship that I am only now beginning to mend.

What I was feeling wasn't the loss of a child. I knew it was just a bunch of cells that never got a chance at life. It was the sense of failure that really got to me. I was young, fit, healthy, intelligent, and yet I couldn't even fulfil the most primitive and basic of female functions.

Once I'd recovered enough to start thinking logically again, I became determined to find the cause behind my miscarriages. Despite the statistics, I felt sure there was a reason for them, and I was going to work it out. This was easier said than done. As callous as it may be, it's difficult to get professional help unless you've had the magical three miscarriages. I wasn't willing to go through that again before anyone would even talk to me. And so I started doing some research of my own.

I'd been seeing an acupuncturist who specialised in

fertility and pregnancy, and between us we began to piece together a theory. My cycle was only three weeks long, and while I seemed to be ovulating around the right time, there were only seven days between that and the arrival of my period—nowhere near long enough for an embryo to implant. I came to believe I had a luteal phase defect, which would mean that in the unlikely event that I could actually conceive, every pregnancy would be doomed to early loss. In addition to this, my acupuncturist believed the problem was in the first half of my cycle, that my eggs were not properly developed before they were released.

Meanwhile, George and I kept trying to get pregnant. He was remarkably good-natured about the whole thing, but it took its toll. In theory, it's every man's dream to have sex on tap, any time of the day, multiple times a week. But in reality, there's nothing much erotic about being propositioned with: 'Let's go, honey, I'm due to ovulate tomorrow!'

I was doing all the things I'd sworn I'd never do—taking my temperature every morning, monitoring cervical mucus, taking note of the slightest changes in my body. I'd become my own worst nightmare. Only those who've been in a similar position can possibly understand the need to be doing *something*.

I finally procured a referral to a specialist at a fertility centre. I shared my theory with her, and she was a little sceptical at first. There has been very little study of luteal phase defects and apparently as a professional you're either a believer or you're not. And she was not. Nevertheless, she proposed that we track my cycle to make sure my body was producing the right chemicals at the right time.

For the next few weeks, I became a human pin cushion, going back to the clinic every three or four days for blood tests. At the end of my usual three-week cycle, I went back for another appointment with the specialist to discuss the next steps.

'There are a few things going on with your cycle,' she began. 'First, you seem to be releasing an egg before it's properly matured. Secondly, you're not producing enough progesterone after you've ovulated, which is why your cycle is so short. There are two things we can do to address these issues.'

As she explained her recommended course of action, a huge weight lifted. It was as if I could breathe properly again for the first time in six months. At last, my instincts had been vindicated. In fact, she told me that my case had cut through her scepticism and made a believer out of her.

Not only had I (and my acupuncturist) been right, but this time I just *knew* it was going to work.

And work it did, immediately. I'm pregnant again now, and this time it's been completely different, right from the start. This time, both of us are ready for it, and excited about it. We've made it past the twelve-week barrier now, and things are looking good. The sight of our baby on the screen at our first ultrasound, wriggling around like a little tadpole, is not something either of us is likely to forget in a hurry.

Every experience shapes us in some way. As difficult as those two miscarriages were at the time, they've made us stronger as a couple. I know we're lucky that our 'problem' turned out to be so easy to solve. I've learnt to trust my instincts, and that a woman usually knows her own body better than any doctor or specialist ever could. I'd like to hope that what happened to us might help other couples.

And I'm sure, in some way, we'll be better parents as a result of what we've been through. We certainly won't be taking any of it for granted.

Rebecca Freeborn has been writing compulsively since she was first able to wield a pen. She has previously published short stories and currently has three novels at varying stages of completion, one of which won her a place on the 2010 Hachette/ Queensland Writer's Centre Manuscript Development Program. Her third pregnancy is still going strong.

The Worry Space
Gillian Freeman

I am standing in Charlie's kinder classroom and his teacher is asking me if my son has trouble taking instruction. She is telling me that when faced with his lunchbox he is unable to decide whether to eat his snack, morning tea or lunch first. It's only the fifth week of his first year of school and I'm thinking that surely this is not abnormal, but I can feel myself starting to panic. I tell myself to breathe, to be brave.

'It just takes him time to settle,' I hear myself saying, but I feel the panic coming, as it always does.

And I know these feelings are not really about the teacher's criticism, or about Charlie's dilemma over the choice between fruit and sandwiches. They are about my two miscarriages.

Charlie is the youngest of three, having a really big sister Millie (nineteen years) and a reasonably big brother Ollie (ten). He is loved by his parents, friends, teachers—everyone. But this adoration comes with a price. He was born after I had two miscarriages in a row and he will probably always inadvertently suffer for this, even if his suffering is only in response to mine.

Like so many women, I have been traumatised by these losses. And it doesn't go away. It doesn't end if you are lucky enough to have another baby, which many of us do. Perhaps I wouldn't be such a basket case if I had known other women—friends and family members—who had also suffered and grieved after a miscarriage. Perhaps I would have benefited from better social networks. Who knows.

At the time I recorded the experience of my third pregnancy and first miscarriage. I wrote about the doctor's visits and prenatal yoga classes. I noted my severe morning sickness and imagined my future as a mother. But, mostly, I wrote about how I was absolutely unprepared when the clinician told me at twelve weeks that there was no baby—only a sac of fluid and other unsavoury things that would have to be removed that afternoon before I got an infection.

I recall the strange reaction I had to this news. Rather than crying and wailing, I felt nothing. I created a kind of imaginary bubble around me. I wrote that instead of giving up, I would treat my miscarriage as a project and bulldoze my way through the problem.

My thinking went something like this:

Day 1: D and C.

Day 2: Grieving for family and friends to see—just enough to make them feel I am human but not too much in case they send me to a psychiatrist or counsellor.

Days 3–28: Try not to cry in front of people and smile nicely when they comment on how tired I look. Be polite and don't respond inappropriately when people give well-meaning advice like, 'It was meant to be' or, 'It's your body's way of getting rid of a bad egg. You wouldn't want to have a ... you know ... baby with a genetic defect.'

This worked to plan and I soon became pregnant again. I raced about telling everyone—even unsuspecting café owners—but was devastated when I started bleeding at a friend's house. We were celebrating my success at becoming a new mother when I dashed to the toilet, only to realise I was miscarrying at five weeks. Again, I made a mental note: *Don't give up. Don't cry. Don't be rude to well-intentioned people.*

When I finally became pregnant for the third time that year (with Charlie), I had the painful experience of going back to the same imaging centre at six weeks to see if there was a heartbeat. I remember sitting on a long bench in the waiting room. Doctors and imaging consultants were coming in and out of the swinging doors. I had read that if there was a heartbeat at six weeks there would only be a two per cent chance of miscarrying. So this moment was critical to my plans and future. I also knew the statistics improved after twelve weeks. So I thought, *Just get through the test and the next six weeks and everything will be fine.*

And on one level it was. I was pregnant. The baby was there and that little darling, Charlie, is still healthy, alive and well today. But this is actually when it all started to go pear-shaped. On knowing I had a real fighting chance, I began to react very strangely. It was during my baby shower that it became really noticable. Everything ought to have been perfect. I had my friends and family around me, and plenty of presents to celebrate the impending birth. On the surface, I couldn't complain. I didn't have gestational diabetes or any of the other ailments that can accompany the third trimester, but I felt sick with dread.

I tried to believe everything was fine, but fear struck at the most unexpected times. Every time I had an ultrasound I had to close my eyes. I couldn't look at the screen that showed my baby and his very healthy heartbeat. My own heart raced at a ridiculous pace and I felt like I was going to be sick. This even happened at my thirty-two-week ultrasound (my choice) when it was blatantly clear there was nothing to worry about.

Then after Charlie was born the panic attacks began. I tried to keep up the polite façade, but my body had other ideas. My brain was trying to control my emotions but my body was shaking and my heart palpitating. I had all the classic symptoms of stress. I was petrified I might lose Charlie. I would jump at the slightest noise. I couldn't breathe if I thought that anything—anything at all—was wrong with him.

This escalated into severe headaches, numbness in my arms and legs, and blurry vision. I tried anti-depressants, sleeping pills, going to a counsellor, and mindfulness techniques—a method of reminding oneself that panic attacks are a physiological response to a scary event and that all we have to do is to breathe while imagining looking at a tiny pea, or something along those lines, as a form of distraction.

I nearly drove one of my best friends insane by panicking about Charlie. We jokingly called this the 'worry space' and laughed that if I didn't worry about Charlie, then surely I would have to worry about something else instead. I wish that were true.

And yet I never felt this way about my other two children, who at one time or another were also singled out at school for parent/teacher discussion. At five, Millie wouldn't—or couldn't—talk to her teachers and was diagnosed with selective mutism by a psychiatrist. The teachers didn't know what to do, so they punished her. For half of her kindie life she sat in the corridor. But this didn't phase me at all; I knew she would grow out of it. And she did.

Similarly, every year up until Year Five Ollie's teachers would comment that he was a slow reader and might need remedial assistance. You would think this would send me into a worrying frenzy, but it didn't. I was a slow reader and so was my husband. I knew Ollie would eventually master it. And he did.

In contrast, Charlie is already a fast reader and talks incessantly to his teachers. Yet I let a little comment about his lunchbox indecisiveness get to me. The miscarriages have changed everything.

In some ways, the panic will never completely go away, although I do practice breathing and mindfulness techniques to keep me sane. There will always be a little bit of fear in relation to mothering a child after a miscarriage, a kind of post-traumatic stress. On the flipside, I couldn't be more in love with Charlie. I long to see him every day, and every night I put him to sleep with a made-up sort-of lullaby. It's a little joke between us that comes out slightly differently each time.

'I love you so much I could eat you,' I say.

'I could eat you more,' Charlie replies, making munching noises.

'I love you more than the whole universe—the stars, the moon, all the planets, the solar system—a million trillion times over.'

'I love you more than the universe spinning around and around and around. I'm putting on my jet-pack and teleporting Doggy and Ollie and Millie and Daddy and Grandma and all my friends and ...'

'Okay, it's bedtime now. Just remember that if you are sad and I'm not there, you can imagine yourself on the moon and I'll meet you there with ...'

'... Doggy and Ollie and Millie and Daddy and ...'

'That's right. It's time to go to sleep now or you'll be too tired for school tomorrow.'

Gillian Freeman is a freelance writer and emerging photographer, currently undertaking a Bachelor of Photography at the Canberra Institute of Technology. She has worked in public relations for the Australian War Memorial and the National Gallery of Australia, and has several degrees in areas including sociology, art history, journalism and professional writing. Gillian has a studio at Gorman House Arts Centre, three gorgeous children and a very handsome husband.

Dissolve

Melinda Small

The monitor flashed to life, humming as it warmed up. The gel was cold and gooey on my stomach, like jelly left sitting out too long after Christmas lunch.

'There we are,' said the doctor as he pointed at the screen.

'Where?' I asked.

'Right there.' He placed his pointer finger on a tiny flashing dot on the screen. 'That's your baby's heartbeat.'

Flickering on the screen in a blur of grey and white was a tiny beeping speck, glowing lightly and then fading, like a firefly. I exhaled slowly, feeling instantly maternal. Watching the glow on the screen, I felt completely content and in love.

Afterwards my husband, Tim, and I drove home, talking about the tiny speck, our baby. We discussed names and cringed at some of the suggestions.

'No way,' I cried indignantly when he suggested Seamus.

'Unlikely,' was his reply when I suggested Ruby.

For now we agreed on Flicker. There was time to settle on a real name later.

Two weeks passed. I felt sick—simultaneously sick and ravenous. My sense of smell became heightened and the familiar fragrances I once enjoyed—like coffee—now signalled the onset of nausea.

I started reading pregnancy books like *What to Expect When You Are Expecting* and announced to Tim that our child was now the size of a grape and was growing tiny fingernails.

We shared the news with family and friends. The sound of popping champagne corks and exclamations of 'I'm going to be a nanny!' filled the house.

At night I lay in bed, my hand gently resting on my slowly expanding stomach. I thought about the baby and the changes it would bring. My own childhood was full of tension and self-deprecation, and I worried that my scars might rub off on this child, a seeping wound unable to be fully closed from one generation to the next. After the fear subsided, I fell asleep with visions of my newborn sleeping softly on my chest.

A few days later I felt a sharp pain. It was accompanied by blood. A giant stain, like a bright red gerbera. I knew it signalled the end.

'There it is,' the doctor said. This time he was pointing at the motionless grey and white matter on the screen. There was no flickering, no tiny glow.

Tim and I looked at the screen, then at each other, and I thought, *My firefly, that perfect little heart, it must have dissolved into mine.*

Melinda Small is the proud mother of two sons, aged six and three. In between their births she had three miscarriages. Melinda is currently studying a Bachelor of Writing at the University of Canberra and divides her time between her sons, work, study, and her love of reading and writing.

What Starts with 'L' and Ends in Chemotherapy?

Sarah Hart

The answer is love, apparently. Who would have thought. Sometimes, for some people, for a very, very small number of potential parents, the story starts with love and ends in chemotherapy.

The first day

The love itself has been there for years, but this particular part of the story started on the tram. On an ordinary day on the way to work.

'I've been thinking about how we want to have kids one day ...'

'Me too! What about it?'

'I was thinking, well, why not now?'

'Me too! I mean, that's exactly what I was thinking!'
'I love you.'
'I love you, too.'

The best day
'Hello, it's Sarah here, I'm just calling to check my blood results?'

'Of course. Let's see ... yep, here we go. Looks like you're about seven or eight weeks. Everything else is perfect. General health is excellent. We'll refer you for an early scan next week so we can confirm those dates, but otherwise looks great. Congratulations.'

The worst day
The screen didn't look right. There was silence. The doctor looked at me and she wasn't smiling. She had a kind face and a professional manner, but she wasn't smiling. She said, 'The important thing to remember is that you know you *can* get pregnant.'

And everything fell apart.

Confusion
Four in the morning. I had a little gap between waves of pain, and I read the post-surgery leaflet again: 'If you pass blood clots bigger than the size of a fifty cent piece, you should go to emergency.' *It's so unfair*, I thought. *I've had the miscarriage, I've had the curette, why can't my body just let me get on with dealing with the rest of it?*

The emergency doctor referred me for another scan, saying she wanted to rule out the possibility there was something left behind after surgery. 'The pathology results show evidence of an abnormal pregnancy,' she said, looking at me as though this should mean something. I nodded. *Of course it was an abnormal pregnancy*, I thought. *If it had been normal, I wouldn't have had a blighted ovum, or whatever it was that other lady said I've had.* I glanced at my file as the doctor was called away. There seemed to be a lot of writing on it. I caught the word 'hydatidiform', but the file was upside down and the word meant nothing to me.

I went home to wait two hours for the scan appointment. I flipped to the back of the baby book for the first time, the part that starts, 'Don't read this unless you have to—the complications described in the following pages are very rare, and most women will never experience them.' I read on, found the word 'hydatidiform' and was horrified. Surely I didn't have this thing? Surely not?

'Didn't they tell you in emergency?' the doctor asked two hours later. 'You've had a molar pregnancy.'

Facts

I'd had a complete molar pregnancy. Or a hydatidiform mole, which is the same thing. It's where conception goes wrong and instead of making a baby, the body makes a placenta and a heap of abnormal cells. You get all the pregnancy symptoms, your hormones say you're pregnant, everything and everyone tells you you're having a baby, but you're not. You're growing a bunch of tumours. You start bleeding a little bit, or a lot, or you have a scan, or surgery, and then the pathology confirms it. You need to get rid of the tumours, or bad things happen. Cancerous things.

Molar pregnancies account for around one in every 1200 pregnancies in Victoria. A specialist centre monitors your urine every week until the tumour marker goes down to zero. You get a letter telling you you're 'satisfactory'. Or you get a call if you're 'not satisfactory'. Ninety per cent of molar pregnancies resolve themselves either through natural miscarriage or surgery. The other ten per cent need further treatment.

The other facts
No one knows about molar pregnancies. You have to explain yourself to everyone. People say horrible things without thinking: 'At least there wasn't a real baby.' You feel like a freak and a failure. If you're in Victoria you spend a lot of time at the Royal Women's Hospital, which is both great and terrible. Great because it means you get the best of care, but terrible because to access that care you have to get in a lift with happily pregnant women and newborns. Worst of all, once you've been diagnosed with a complete molar pregnancy, you can't try to get pregnant again for twelve months after the tumour marker hits zero. Twelve whole months.

Waiting
We entered a weird no-man's-land. Instead of finding out the baby's sex at the start of what would have been my second

trimester, my partner and I were watching the post and trying not to terrify ourselves by reading too much on the internet. Instead of comparing bumps with my more successfully pregnant work colleague, I was sneaking around trying not to cry. Instead of spreading the good news, we were having to explain, over and over again, the implications of a disease we'd only just found out existed.

Two days after receiving a letter saying my second to latest test was satisfactory, I got the call. My latest test was not satisfactory. The tumours were growing and I now had persistent gestational trophoblastic disease. I was one of the ten per cent.

Chemotherapy
There was a seventy-five per cent chance further surgery wouldn't work and I would have to have chemotherapy anyway. So I started on methotrexate chemotherapy, which is injections every other day. You don't really get used to the smell of blood, or the crippling cramping pains, or hanging out in the day chemo room, or mouth ulcers, or having to explain your weird disease to everyone, or not having an end date to the treatment. But you can manage it. What I couldn't manage was the chest pain, which started just after the second cycle finished.

It crept up. It was a bit hard to breathe, then a bit painful to breathe. So I went to emergency and they gave me some drugs and told me not to worry.

It was pleuritic chest pain, a rare side effect of methotrexate, and it got worse and worse over the next two weeks. For most people it remains mild. For a tiny proportion it becomes something else altogether, and by the middle of my third cycle of chemo I was back in emergency. I'd never known pain like it. I was being knifed in the back with every breath. Even the smallest movement was painful, and the big movements, especially the ones I couldn't control, like throwing up, were torture. I couldn't keep pills down, so they ended up giving me a lot of morphine, which at least spaced me out a bit, even if it didn't actually stop the pain. I spent a week in hospital.

A lovely nurse caught me crying when I was finally on the mend and gave me a journal article about the chest pain side effect. It was reassuring to know that I wasn't entirely alone. Although I found it difficult to count my blessings lying there in the complex care ward with way too much time to think. I could see out the window into the ward on the neighbouring wing. I don't know which one it was exactly, but it was something to do with birth. Through two panes of glass and five stories of air I got to watch couple after couple wander into view in the lounge area holding their babies and balloons and overnight bags.

You can't manage that sort of pain.

Statistics
About one in 1200 pregnancies is a molar pregnancy. About one-third of those are complete molar pregnancies. About ten per cent of that one-third develop persistent and/or metastatic characteristics and need methotrexate chemotherapy. About twenty per cent of that ten per cent experience some degree

of chest pain. About fifteen per cent of that twenty per cent experience such severe pain they need to be taken off methotrexate and put on something else.

I've tried to work out the overall odds, but it's meaningless in the end. Because the odds of it all happening to me turned out to be one hundred per cent.

Things I had to say

There are some things you never dream you'll have to say, so you don't prepare, and then you choke:

I'm miscarrying ...

I have an appointment with the oncologist ...

My psychologist says ...

I can't, I have chemo that day ...

We aren't allowed to try again for twelve months ...

It's all right, it's highly curable ...

It didn't feel all right. I felt like my body had become a battleground, with the molar cells on one side and modern medicine on the other. I was in the middle, having to keep up with the collateral damage and act as interpreter. I didn't want to be in a battle, or interpret, or be highly curable, or know what goes on in the complex care ward. I just wanted to curl up with my original grief. I lost our baby. I lost our baby. I lost our baby ...

The home stretch

I was switched to second line chemotherapy, Actinomycin D. Hooked up to a machine for a couple of hours a day, five days per week, then a week off. It was exhausting. I got pretty sick, lost a lot of hair (but not all of it), struggled with drug-induced insomnia. But no more chest pain, no more bleeding and finally—*finally*—an end date. I finished chemotherapy in mid-December, just in time to be reasonably upright for Christmas.

Now

I'm okay now. I go in for monthly blood tests to check whether it's coming back. It probably won't, according to my oncologist, and I probably won't have another molar pregnancy. The chances are tiny. Which feels meaningless (see 'Statistics' above).

I've learned a heap of things I already knew, but didn't really know. That I can endure more than I ever imagined when there is no other choice. That I can fail spectacularly. That it's almost impossible to feel optimistic when you're in pain. That my partner is the most wonderful man in the world. That we really, really do want children, enough to accept that the same thing might happen again, and still plan to try.

This is part of our story now. These words I've written, they are all true, and they are all about me, about us, about our attempt to start a family. I never dreamt it would turn out like this, and I still can't quite believe it has. I'm hoping we can somehow fit it all in to our lives without too much long-term damage. I'm hoping it turns out to be just a sad and surreal footnote to our real story—the one that starts with love and ends in love. I'm hoping.

Sarah Hart has had short fiction and opinion pieces published in a hotchpotch of newspapers, journals and magazines, including The Age, twenty600, Lip, Capital Magazine, The Canberra Times *and* Horsewyse. *This story is the hardest thing she has ever tried to write, about the hardest thing that has ever happened to her.*

A Blanket of Words
Heidi Silberman

I stood in my classroom, waiting for nine o'clock, a silly smile slipping across my face. Graffiti scrawled on a desk caught the attention of my fingers and I traced it distractedly, willing time to go faster. I jumped when the bell finally rang. The discordant voices of teenage boys filled the hallways, their laughter reverberating throughout the old building. My Year Sevens bustled into the room, removing caps, tucking in shirts and pulling up socks. I tapped the desk impatiently. The noise died down and I called the roll. I couldn't wait any longer, I simply couldn't hold it in.

'I have some news.'

They looked at me, most of them, some still fiddled with their bags or tried to continue their conversations without me noticing. But I didn't care, not today.

'I'm having a baby. I'm pregnant.'

They glanced at each other with looks I didn't understand. 'We'll tell the whole year group by recess,' one boy said, setting a challenge to the rest. I didn't believe him, but they did it.

In the corridor on the way to class I was approached by another teacher.

'Are you pregnant?' he asked

'Yes!' I beamed.

He looked at my skinny belly, evidently confused. 'How far along are you?'

'Four weeks!'

I was ecstatic. He was concerned. 'And you told the boys?'

'Yes!'

'But, what if—why are you telling everyone now? What if something happens?'

I studied him briefly. Older than me, married and with kids of his own, I thought he should understand. 'Then I'll share that with them too.'

I wanted everyone to know my good news, but I also wanted them to know my bad news, if there was to be any. My father had died only a few months earlier and I had been unable to carry that grief alone. I had needed to talk, to share my experience with friends and family, even with those of my students who asked. If indeed something happened, and I lost this baby, I would need people to know.

Nothing did 'happen'. Our beautiful Joshua was born in due time and his sister Rebekah came along two years later. When I became pregnant a third time, Dave and I were thrilled and again told everyone. The symptoms were identical to my first two pregnancies—nausea, sore breasts, constant weeing. These were things I didn't share with others.

I was exactly twelve weeks along when I noticed a little bleeding. I spoke to my mum on the phone, nervously admitting, 'It just doesn't feel right.'

I looked up the books, which said it could be normal, but may not be. Sleep came fearfully that night.

In the morning I saw my GP, leaving the kids with my concerned mother while Dave went to work. By now I was also feeling immense pressure above my pelvis. I hoped and prayed this was normal, that everything would be all right, but fear grew when the pressure intensified into an ache. The doctor encouraged me to go home and rest, but twenty-four hours later she sent me to the antenatal ward of the local hospital.

The ache was turning to pain. I had read so many pregnancy books and each one only mentioned miscarriage in passing—as a possibility, a statistic. There were no details. Not one described what it would be like. I wouldn't have enjoyed reading about it, but now—stuck in the middle of one—I wished I had some idea, some knowledge, something to prepare me.

The pain was unnervingly familiar. Wave upon wave enveloped me before I realised the truth: these were contractions. My mind fought the pain while my body calmly remembered and told me lies. *This is good pain. Work with the pain, you'll have a beautiful baby at the end of it. It's all for a good cause, there will be a happy ending. The baby is coming!* But when the baby came there was no joy, no happy ending.

That weekend we travelled to Sydney for the funeral of Dave's grandfather, Lloyd. There, grieving relatives and friends shared memories of Lloyd, celebrated his life and comforted each other. I wanted to scream: 'What about my baby? Will anyone talk about my baby? Where was my baby's life? When was my baby's funeral?' I wanted to talk. I needed to. And over lunch, while everyone spoke about Lloyd, my beautiful sister-in-law Peggy listened as I shared my story.

Driving home I looked forward to playgroup the next week. I had walked the paths of parenthood with these women for four years. We had struggled together and celebrated milestones, but none of them had suffered a miscarriage. Again I needed someone's ears. I needed to release my tears and receive their comfort. But as I walked through the doorway I realised how close I was to drowning in this sea of grief. I waited for someone to throw me a lifebuoy. These mums looked up, tentatively smiling. Someone said hello. Someone else took the craft activity I had brought and set it up. I sank a little and felt the waves pushing me. People talked to Josh and Bekky. But no one asked how I was.

As the waters threatened to overtake me, Janette took me aside. Perhaps she would be my rescuer. She told me how sad she was, and I felt myself being lifted up. My tears began to escape; at last it was safe to talk. But then she turned back to the group and the moment was gone. I fell back into the water, the waves higher than ever.

I understood that no one knew what to say, but all I needed was a question, one person to ask, 'How are you?' I waited. I was sinking fast and still no one gave me permission. I hadn't wanted to make anyone uncomfortable, now I was the uncomfortable one. I did craft with the children and somehow made it through the two hours until we said goodbye. I strapped the kids in the car, put my head on the steering wheel and wept.

I had recently begun attending another playgroup in preparation for Josh starting preschool. We had only been a few times so I didn't know these women well. The leader rang to see where I had been for the last few weeks. I told her, she listened. She had experienced a miscarriage too. The next week at the group another mum told me in detail her story of losing a baby. Her loss had happened a few years earlier, but was as raw as ever. As she spoke I felt her pain pressing on mine. The tale went on. Her tears emerged, along with anger and other emotions. I didn't know if I could cope with her grief as well as mine but it was obvious she needed to talk. I understood the need to be heard, and clearly she had not yet found enough people willing to listen. So I obliged, even though it hurt.

That was eight years ago. Even now it seems that each time I speak of my loss, there is another woman with a miscarriage story to tell. There is another mother with hidden grief she can only share with someone she knows will understand. Often she had lost her baby before announcing her pregnancy. Suddenly she was empty and had to find other ways to grieve. Now, years later, perhaps having had other children, she jumps at the opportunity to tell her story. We sneak together into that locked room in her heart. We pick up our babies and hold them the only way we can, wrapped in a blanket of words. When we have finished, the room is a little brighter, the curtains open to let in a little more light and this time we won't lock the door as we leave.

Heidi Silberman is a Christian who lives in Canberra with her husband and four gorgeous children. She is a performer and tutor for Impro ACT. As a qualified teacher she has taught improvised theatre to primary, high school and adult students. When the house is quiet she loves to write about her children on her blog, Postcards from Planet Chaos, at http://cupofteatime. wordpress.com

Black Holes—The Art of Losing Babies
Anne Myers

Bored now that his patient was asleep, the anaesthetist eyed me, the new nurse, and started chatting. It came out that I was soon to be forty. He could not believe it. 'No way,' he said, wearing his theatre cap like he thought he was George Clooney though he was probably closer in age to George's father. 'There's no way you look forty.' He paused a moment. 'Ah,' he said, 'but do you have children?'

'No,' I replied, my standard answer for a first-day-on-the-job standard question.

He pointed his finger at me in triumph. 'I knew it, I *knew* it, that's why you don't look forty.'

I wanted to take his George Clooney cap and tourniquet his neck and explain that if he only knew the half of it I should look at least eighty, but I didn't. I blushed a little, smiled as if I had not a care in the world and put up another bag of saline.

In my twenties, babies were good in theory, my ovaries twitched every now and then but mostly lay quiet. And there were women artists I gravitated towards purely because they had no children. Frida Kahlo, Georgia O'Keefe, Virginia Woolf. How I admired them with their days of unhindered creativity, their other-worldliness, so far removed from my life as a nurse in inner Melbourne. I longed to live my life as these women had done. I wanted to be them. And not having children suited me fine.

Fifteen years later, the irony is not lost on me as they slip back into my life. Not that they ever really left, but the gravitational pull has strengthened. I have sought them out again now that a life without children is right in my face and I have changed my mind. They have become my unofficial mentors in this baby-making business. Or perhaps I'm bringing them in early, absorbing them prophylactically, so they'll be there for me when my uterus shuts up shop.

On my wall hangs Imogen Cunningham's photograph of Frida Kahlo. It is a beautiful portrait. She sits in her traditional Mexican peasant dress, serene, unsmiling, dignified. Underneath her clothes lies a body of scars. Her face reads pain. Frida had always wanted children. Unfortunately, a bus accident in Mexico City as a teenager physically prevented her from ever carrying one to term and she was advised by doctors to forgo any future pregnancies. Four miscarriages later and her husband, Diego Rivera 'forbade her to conceive again'. So she kept monkeys and dogs, cats, parrots, doves, an eagle, a deer, the odd lover or two, and painted her loss in all its bloodiness.

Georgia O'Keefe also wanted children. She had cared

for her younger sister often and found the experience gratifying though the responsibility for someone else's life frightened her. Through self-interest or concern for her welfare, her husband, the photographer Alfred Steiglitz, ensured she never became a mother. He had lost his sister during childbirth, and his only daughter from a previous relationship had been diagnosed with schizophrenia soon after the birth of her son and he blamed himself for her mental illness. He would not allow Georgia to have children. Besides, he was focused on her developing as a painter. Georgia acceded to his request.

And lastly, Virginia Woolf, she also wanted to become a mother. It was Leonard Woolf who felt her mental and physical strength would never be able to cope with the demands of children. Perhaps he was right. And so she begat no babies and went to an early grave childless.

Their work outlived them, not their bloodline. And if it wasn't for the work they created I would not be writing about them in the first place. It is the fact they never had children that brings them back into my life, a path not of their, or my, choosing. It is difficult to say how these three women's lives may have developed if they had all given birth to living offspring. How might their bodies of work have been different? Many might be pleased they never had children if that meant their art was more voluminous than otherwise. Back then, I thought I understood their pain, all that painted blood oozing out between Frida's legs, but what did I know?

I look at these women with their reasons for not having children and I want to write about my own reasons but I have none. My uterus was never punctured with a metal handrail on an overcrowded rickety bus, my husband is not in the habit of making decisions on my behalf, and I have never suffered from depression. Sometimes I wish I was still in the camp of not wanting children and I envy women who know this with conviction. I wish I was older so it would be behind me and I could plan my life without the burden (and yes it has become that) of hoping for a child, but I am smack bang in the twilight years of my fertility and the end seems way over there.

There is no reason why I can't have children. Nothing proven. And yet I harbour the deepest of black holes. It has nothing to do with space and discovery. There's a black hole in my gut where a baby should be. I should be anatomically correct and use the term *uterus* but *gut* bears more grunt when I say it out loud and I'm in the mood for that kind of out-loud-gutsy speak. These days, my husband and I are becoming experts in the art of losing babies. It's not forgetfulness and a matter of finding them again, they're just not hanging around.

There are no names, no funerals to attend, no yearly remembrances, just vague days spent lying on a trolley with a fat pad between my legs as bits of the promised land seep out. There's a small quilt-for-one given to me by kind volunteers, a small angel patchworked into one corner, and there's been plenty of pretending to be asleep in order to avoid the sympathetic gaze when well-intentioned pastoral care workers sidle up next to my trolley.

Perhaps if there was a baby crying in the next room there might be no need to write this and all those years of angst would somehow be diminished, wrapped up in the delight of a new life. But there isn't a baby. And we can't know if there will ever be. That's what makes it so difficult and what keeps us going back, just like the addicts—one more time, just one more time.

I wanted this piece to start out matter-of-fact, beginning with the latest miscarriage, three days ago. The kind of morning it was, how much traffic was about, the easy park right across the road from our appointment, how I could hear the rain on the roof that morning, my husband next to me wide awake listening to the radio through his earphones. We would arrive at the hospital with one minute to spare, jumping across the raised tram tracks and narrowly avoiding sprained ankles or a direct hit with the city-bound tram. There would be hints of spring everywhere and no more so than with myself, anticipating the smiles and contentment of seeing our baby's heartbeat for the first time. Then seeing the familiar black hole. But I don't want sentiment or sympathy, there is enough of that in my life already.

Perhaps people don't even want to read about losing babies. Or trying to have them. It's a tough one. Like having a newborn, not having a newborn is intensive and tiring and can easily become the main focus in your life. Yet there is nothing physical to show for it. No photographs to pass around, nothing to peek at. There are plenty of impersonal stories in the tabloids; the financial burden of infertility treatment complete with a photograph of a sad-looking couple having used their life savings for no end result. Are we that couple?

I have wanted to write about losing babies before now but mostly the energy has not been there. Living through the experience, there is barely enough energy for the disappointments, let alone writing about them, and often I would rather be thinking or reading about something less depressing.

But here we are, a group that very much exists. We're the group who live a double life, who are happy when our friends become pregnant before excusing ourselves to go to the bathroom to take deep breaths and avoid looking at ourselves in the mirror. The group who run hot and cold with others depending on where we are at in our cycle (and we humbly apologise). One moment pleased to be offering up any news, the next eyes downcast in dread of being spoken to. And I despise being seen as this kind of person, to be labelled as the one who's having trouble having kids, but some primitive part in me behaves in ways that I fail to recognise as myself. It is a world not of my choosing and often it chooses its own reactions for me.

Yet some days I am confident to wear this badge, when the drugs have all worn off and my brain has returned back to earth, to be the spokeperson for all those who do not speak openly about it. I want to speak about it as others speak about their babies sleeping habits, or the latest cute little thing their baby is doing. I want to speak freely, to validate my life as this person trying to have a child. I am not ashamed. I am where I am. I have as much validity as the woman holding a new baby, believe it or not. This is my life. But on certain days it comes down to this—I want what she's got—and then I'm left numbly sitting in my room trying to make sense of it all.

I lie on the trolley, the condom-covered probe in my vagina as the sonographer hones in on our little baby. There it is on the screen. And she kindly describes everything in detail. 'There's its head, and there's its arms and legs ...' and on and on she goes.

My husband and I smile at each.

'... and there's its heart, but unfortunately it's not beating.'

What? Has she really taken this approach, giving us a detailed description of our little baby only to tell us that it's dead?

We head back to the waiting room, the usual intensified surrounds of prams and pregnant bellies in our faces.

I get online and drift into chat rooms where other women give detailed resumes of their gynaecological lives, where they're at with things, how stressed they are, reading about the exquisite pain of continuously waiting for egg collection, for embryo transfer, for pregnancy tests, but the intensity of anguish en masse is unbearable.

It can be a trap hanging out with people in the same situation. While supportive, it may end up becoming burdensome. A fear arises in anticipation of another's pregnancy, a guilty resentment that they sealed the deal, and have now moved into a different world, all the time wishing secretly it was you who was leaving that world behind. And it has been me before, even if only for a few months I too have dared to look forward into the future, to dream of a family. When each pregnancy results in no baby, you begin to believe this can be the only outcome and you talk yourself into this outcome because it is the only way to cope when it does fail.

I am going on holidays, I tell an older collegue at work. She asks me if I have any children. That same question again and again, an innocent enough question, a question that will continue to be asked until the day I die.

'No,' I reply. Even in saying this simple word of two letters, I find there are so many ways to say it, all the different tonal inflections depending on the day, the mood, the person. No. No. No.

'Holidays? You shouldn't be needing any holidays if you don't have children,' she says, laughing.

And so the conversations continue.

It might be easy to imagine how sad our lives must be throughout all this. And, yes, of course there has been sadness. But life does move on around us and we're on board most of the time. We are grateful we are soulmates. It gets us through the tough gigs. We have a great life together. And we have found the humour in it all. Take our latest black hole. The sonographer takes a picture, places it in an envelope and hands it to me like a present. I actually thank her. We sit in a cafe afterwards, not wanting to go home, not wanting to restart our lives again just yet, as if nothing has happened. So we drive to the Botanical Gardens. We park the car opposite the shrine and running near us on the outside running track is the biggest group of mums and prams I have ever seen, some kind of aerobics class. They stop right in front of us and start swinging their legs side-to-side using their prams as the ballet barre. We have to laugh. There is no escaping life, it is everywhere. The gardens swallow us whole, its lush green the perfect antidote.

And so I continue to write and I can only hope Frida, Georgia and Virginia are with me in spirit, pushing me to excel at my great love. I know a life without children is becoming more likely with each passing year. I know that that life is a good life and will be and has been so far a rich and fulfilling one. I say I am ready for that kind of life, but as each cycle begins, as I swallow the oestrogen and progesterone and the hormones chill me out, as that addict in me comes to the fore, I fall in love again with the idea of being a mother.

Anne Myers is a writer whose work has appeared in Southerly, Meanjin, The Age, The Death Mook *and on Radio National.*

Not Talia

Melissa Ferguson

Brad and I are the only people in the windowless waiting room. I flick through a glossy magazine and glimpse evening gowns, high heels, lips, eyes and shiny hair.

'Melissa Ferguson?'

I stand and wipe my sweaty hands on my jeans. We follow the sonographer into a dim ultrasound room.

'You did my last ultrasound,' I say. My stomach clenches into a small hard ball.

She scans my face like a passport inspector. 'Was it a miscarriage?'

'Yes.' I lie down on the bed and pinch the stiff sheets between my thumb and forefinger.

'So how many weeks are you now?'

'Twelve weeks yesterday.'

'And everything's been okay so far?'

'Seems to be. I've been very nauseous though.'

'That's a good sign.' She picks up the probe and adjusts her seat. 'Well let's have a look then.'

Ten months ago my period was late. I knew because I'd been marking the days on the calendar and calculating ovulation dates. I ate two packets of sour cream and sweet chilli chips, one after the other. Beneath my bellybutton things felt different. My uterus was kind of itchy, as though a layer of fur had grown inside it.

I dipped a pregnancy test stick into a cup of my wee and left it on the bathroom sink. Brad sat on the couch reading a surfing magazine. He looked up at me and raised his eyebrows.

'Ten minutes,' I said, and folded some washing.

The second blue line was faint, like a photocopy of a photocopy, but it was there. We were having a baby.

A week later we were in New Zealand on holidays. On our first morning in Queenstown we awoke to a clear blue sky. We had two weeks of holiday ahead of us and the hope for a wonderful future cocooned inside me. We found a busy café with tables spilling out into the sunlight. Brad had poached eggs on toast. Pregnancy hadn't made me nauseous, so I ordered pancakes with berries.

'You know, I think it's a girl. What do you think of Talia for a name?' I said.

'Yeah, I like it.'

After breakfast I walked through the café to the toilet. In the kitchen, cutlery and plates clattered, steam hissed and black-clad waitresses yelled their orders. When I returned all I could hear was my heart thumping in my ears.

'What's wrong?' Brad asked.

'It's probably nothing ... just a bit of brown blood.'

'How much?'

'Only a little bit. I'm pretty sure spotting isn't unusual during pregnancy. I'm sure my body knows what it's doing.'

I'm the kind of person who waits to see if a headache will go away by itself before I resort to aspirin or paracetamol. I trust my body, I look after it and I expect it to return the favour.

'Just keep an eye on it.'

Brad and I rented a campervan and headed toward Milford Sound. In a newsagency in Taupo I picked up a pregnancy book and a copy of *Charlotte's Web* for Talia, as a sign of faith in her survival.

Later that day we sat on a windswept beach and ate fish and chips. I pulled my cardigan tight around me and opened the pregnancy book. I comforted myself with reassuring words about bleeding in pregnancy and skipped over the warnings that any prolonged bleeding should be assessed by a doctor.

Over the next ten days I crossed my fingers and took a deep breath whenever I visited the toilet. Sometimes, when my underpants and the toilet paper were clear, I thought that must be the end of it. Other times a spot of blood would knock the wind out of me like a punch to the stomach. I started visiting the toilet almost hourly, just to check. I didn't mention anything to Brad. I didn't want to ruin his holiday, and as long as I was silent I was still a woman expecting a baby.

On the second last day of our trip I sat in a stall in the

camping ground toilet block with a pregnancy test stick in my hand. I imagined that the blue line would only appear if a tiny heartbeat persisted in my womb. With closed eyes I tapped my feet against the concrete floor and counted, 'one-cat-and-dog, two-cat-and-dog …' all the way to five hundred. I opened my eyes. Two blue lines. Surely that meant the spotting would stop in coming days.

It didn't. It got heavier.

On the flight home Brad and I sat side-by-side, facing forwards as though in a confessional, and I told him about the spotting.

'I think you should see a doctor,' he said.

I nodded and looked out the window. Things weren't going to sort themselves out.

The GP was a middle-aged woman with spectacles and curly hair. By her calculations I was ten weeks pregnant. I wanted her to test a sample of my body fluids or apply an instrument to my belly or use her physician's intuition and tell me my baby was okay. Instead she booked an ultrasound for the following day.

Sitting in the radiology centre waiting room my bladder was a balloon about to burst. I still had a tiny hope the sonographer would find Talia's heartbeat and reassure me she was perfectly healthy and that I would be a mum in thirty weeks time.

The sonographer led me into the ultrasound room. She applied the probe to my abdomen and searched the screen. After a couple of minutes of silence she said, 'I'm going to have to try vaginally.'

'Okay.'

'You can empty your bladder first. Then take off your jeans and put this gown on.'

When I sat down on the toilet there was a gush of blood. My stomach jumped up into my chest. I returned clutching my jeans in front of me like a shield. 'I'm bleeding quite a lot now.'

'That's okay we'll have a look anyway,' she said gently.

She took a couple of pictures. I peered at indecipherable white images within the slice-shaped area on the screen.

'I'm afraid there's no heartbeat. The foetus looks about six weeks old. The bleeding will get heavier now, until the foetus has been passed and your uterus is empty.'

I blinked back my tears and bit my lip to stop it from quivering. My dead baby had been inside me for four weeks.

'Don't worry. The same thing happened to me once. You'll have another baby.'

The sonographer was so kind I wanted to thank her, but I couldn't speak.

After the dark examination room the sunlight blinded me. On my way home fat tears fell and pooled above my breastbone. Brad came home from work early and we sat on the couch together and sobbed.

The next day at the hospital emergency department a young doctor pulled a curtain around our cubicle and sat on the chair across from Brad and me. She advised us that current hospital policy was to let the uterus shed its lining unassisted and only perform a curette if there was anything remaining that might cause infection.

'This must be hard. Only a short time ago you must have been thinking about what it would be like to have a baby.' She gave me a sympathetic look.

'When can I start trying to get pregnant again?'

'Wait until after your next period. Just so we know everything has returned to normal.'

After a week of medically certified grieving time I returned to work and pretended it had never happened. I kept thinking, *I shouldn't be feeling this bad. Much worse things have happened to other people.* My brother Stephen died when he was seven months old. Some sort of throat infection. When I was young my friends would ask about the photo of the newborn with tightly clenched fists and plastic hospital tags around his wrists. 'That's Stephen. He died when he was a baby,' I would say. We'd look at the photo in solemn awe for a couple of seconds and then return to playing jacks or choreographing dance routines. That was a tragedy—the death of a child who had been carried for forty weeks, given birth to, cared for and loved for seven months. Talia was just a barely formed bundle of cells.

I attributed my grief to hormones. *Nature's way of ensuring the propagation of the species*, my inner biologist said. The only thing I wanted was to get pregnant again. Every month I was disappointed when my period arrived with the punctuality of a dreaded utility bill. Everywhere I looked I saw smug women, round and ripe as watermelons, and I wondered why it was so easy for everyone else. Looking back I realise I had no idea what those other women had gone through. Maybe they had lost children or had miscarriages or undergone gruelling fertility treatments.

After hearing about my miscarriage, a couple of people told me about theirs. I hadn't heard these stories before. I suppose I wouldn't have understood. I'd have felt sorry for them but I wouldn't have felt empathy. I would have thought, *It won't ever happen to me.*

My friend Amanda and I met for lunch one Sunday in a colourful café with mismatched furniture. I looked and felt terrible. I'd just got my period again.

'How are things?' Amanda asked.

'Okay, I suppose. Still not pregnant. It's becoming a bit of an obsession. I don't know why it's taking so long.'

'Oh. I was hoping you would be ... because I am ... pregnant. I'm due in November.'

'That's great. I thought you weren't ready for a baby?' I smiled and raised the pitch of my voice the way people did when they were happy.

'Yeah well, it was a bit of an accident. But then I had a little bit of brown blood last week and I was really devastated when I thought I might lose the baby.'

'What happened with the blood?'

'It stopped by itself. I had an ultrasound and the baby was fine.'

'That's what happened to me you know ... brown blood.' *How come* my *bleeding didn't stop?*

I stopped marking the dates of my period and possible ovulation dates on my calendar and forgot about the whole thing.

Early in September the estimated due date for Talia's

birth passed. Soon after, I realised I hadn't had my period for a while. And my breasts were sore. And I was eating a lot of sour cream and sweet chilli chips.

I put the pregnancy test stick on the bathroom sink and looked at my watch. I looked back and there was already a vivid blue line. *What if it happens again? What if all my pregnancies end in early miscarriage?* I just needed to make it to twelve weeks with a heartbeat.

Brad and I watch the grainy image on the screen. The shape of a tiny creature, with a big head, lying on its back appears.

'There's the heartbeat,' she says.

Brad squeezes my hand. Tears prick my eyes.

'The foetus looks well-formed and the right size for twelve weeks,' she says.

The baby waves its arms and kicks its feet as though trying to push away the sound waves invading its dark cave. I can see its head and its jawbone and the curve of its spine. It's not Talia. It's her little brother or sister and they have a powerful, beating heart.

Before becoming a mother of two Melissa Ferguson's biography would have reflected her love of travel and live music, and her career as a cancer-fighting scientist. Now she likes a cup of tea and a piece of chocolate after the kids have gone to bed. Melissa is working on a memoir about her difficult and surprising transformation into 'Mum'.

If the Blood had Come
Karen Andrews

Vanishing Twin Syndrome.

Take a moment to fully comprehend that phrase. It sounds ludicrous—as if a twin could just vanish! But mine did. And even though it's been over five years since my baby disappeared, I'm still asking myself questions.

I'd never heard of Vanishing Twin Syndrome or its acronym (VTS) until my second pregnancy. We were introduced during an ultrasound only seconds after I joked with my obstetrician that I hoped only one baby would be present, please! Like a metronome, back and forth, went his sonic-reading wand.

And then it stopped. As did my heart.

He traced a circle with his finger on the monitor, circling the blighted ovum. He explained, 'This actually happens quite a lot.'

For him, perhaps.

I always thought miscarriages involved bleeding. This was the instruction I took from movies and television. A trilogy of events—a look of pain, a protective hand over the pubis, a glimpse of red—indicated what was happening. But my miscarriage *did* happen without bleeding, and years later I'm still having trouble processing my feelings. My internal spirit level wobbles daily.

That day my questioning began. I wondered if all the scans and statistics weren't just a tenuous attempt to predict the future. I wanted to be assured that the remaining baby was well (he was, and remains so to this day), but ultimately no procedure could make that promise. At the same time I wondered about my doctor's warning that I may not bleed, that instead I would in all likelihood reabsorb the foetal tissues.

Where was the funeral, the reclamation to dust? None of the usual rituals of goodbye were available, so instead I became a living mausoleum. If the tissues were reabsorbed, what became of them? Were they recycled as hair that I would later cut or fingernails I would chew?

In my confused state I turned to an online parenting forum I was a member of and posted my raw thoughts. I was sad, yes, but also … relieved. I already had a one year old daughter and the prospect of three children under the age of two was positively frightening. Logistical concerns first, guilt later.

This guilt quickly arrived on a wave of disgust and ire that was returned to me, in comment form, by one member of the forum who I considered a friend. *How dare you be so insensitive to say that in front of other women who you know are having fertility issues*, I was told. *You realise they'd swap places in an instant? That they would be grateful for the remaining baby?*

Other friends jumped to my defence, yet I also heard that my name was being whispered, via private messages, in none too flattering terms. I left the forum after apologising for any offence I might have caused.

So I mourned alone. I remained relieved, and yet I mourned. On quiet afternoons when I could stand to face learning more about VTS I turned to the internet. But it was to little avail. Pregnancy books don't often mention it, or if they do it's in footnoted form. And yet, even if entire chapters were to be found, if hidden internet hyperlinks magically revealed themselves, I doubt they would tell me what I secretly want to know. Were you a boy or a girl? Where are you now?

If the blood had come, perhaps that might have helped. If the blood had come, the ghosts might not have taken up residence in my heart.

But if the blood had come, I might have lost both babies. Or myself in the grief.

As I look back on that day when my baby apparently vanished, I now know what I wanted. For my doctor to say, 'I'm sorry.' For him to hand me an information pamphlet or give me a number to call. But I was offered no consolation.

Instead I walk around in an anachronistic jumble. I like building blocks for this reason. While I play with my children I lay them out to spell 'love' and rub my fingers along the cube edges. I rub my stomach too, for old time's sake. I close my eyes and remember.

Karen Andrews is an author and award-winning poet and short story writer. She runs a successful blog at Miscellaneous Mum (www.miscmum.com), and is a publisher at Miscellaneous Press. She is quite keen on old Hollywood themed coffee-table books and macaroons.

The Detour

Christine Darcas

In 1974, at thirteen years old, I decided that I would never be a stay-at-home mother. I might get married, even have a family, but that would not limit my drive to use my mind and develop my potential through a career. I made this decision with the naïve certainty that with enough determination and hard work I could navigate my future—including the arrival of children—on my terms.

I grew up in America through the full swing of the women's liberation movement. The chants of angry women wielding placards and punching the air with fists filled our living room on the evening news. The day of my decision, I attended a French class at a local university with my thirty-four-year-old mother who was determined to complete the undergraduate degree she had dutifully abandoned at nineteen to become a housewife. While I cringed beside her in my green-pleated school uniform, she sat up front and fluttered her fingers to answer, correctly, nearly every question the professor asked.

Roughly fifteen years younger, her female classmates chewed gum, twirled long, unkempt hair and passed quips beneath their breath. Adolescent confusion consumed me. I was embarrassed by my mother's age and teacher's-pet eagerness, but proud of her, too. She had guts to be there, and she was there, I realised, because she needed to be. Cooped up at home with three kids, she had come to stalk the house like a caged cheetah. And, damn, she was *smart*. For the first time, I understood that by becoming a stay-at-home mother, my mum had squandered her potential. It was a choice that struck me as an enormous mistake, and one that I was determined not to repeat.

My plan proceeded well enough. I graduated from a strong liberal arts university in America, then became an aid worker in Chad, embracing opportunities beyond the grasp of so many women in my mother's generation. In Chad, I met a young Frenchman named François-Xavier. Working in the countryside brittle with drought or the mortar-pocked capitol of N'djamena, we crossed and crisscrossed until I came to know, then adore, the steady, intelligent and amusing man beneath his quiet reserve. But while my feelings for him deepened, my resilience to the poverty, sick children and general civil viciousness burned down and exhausted. I left Chad, and François joined me.

Neither one of us was preoccupied with children; during our first five years together we rarely discussed them. We wed, went to business school and revved up careers in New York City where I made the final cut for a marketing position within the soap and detergent division of a large multinational. It was a stimulating and rigorous existence. I was expected to adhere to a reliably driven work ethic, to persevere into the night and over weekends, take flights at the crack of dawn to attend meetings in distant cities, then fly right back to arrive in the office bright and early the next morning. To deliver anything less risked jeopardising my career. Working part-time wasn't even an option.

Then I started to notice the babies.

They snuck up on me. As I queued at the pharmacy, one reached out from her pram and brushed her fingertips along my calf. I swung around to see her peering up at me, her expression a combination of apprehension and cheeky smile. On one of my business trips, a harried mum in an airport terminal asked me to hold her grizzling baby boy while she deftly mixed a bottle of formula. I grasped him under his armpits while he bounced on my tailored suit lap. Up and down, up and down, he sprung on his pudgy legs, his little bare feet planted firmly on my thighs, screeching with glee as if he was just discovering the promise of his own strength.

I was ready. More than ready—I actually *yearned* to have a child. It was as if dormant instincts had awoken within me, creating an urging, consuming need.

Foolishly, I had never doubted that I could have children. I was strong, I was able. I presumed that I could manage a family and career. According to the women covering the television news of my youth, it was something I was *supposed* to do. Anything else compromised my ability, was a declaration of weakness that I couldn't do both. The fact that I fell pregnant the first month we tried reinforced my self-perception of strength.

The day I found out, I dangled my positive pregnancy test in front of my dazed husband. François had only just started a new job, was still carving his niche in an equally competitive environment. But his face broke into a huge grin. So what if we lived in a one-bedroom flat in a hugely expensive metropolis? So what if we already lived on a strict budget? We had always managed. I had always managed. Anyway, I felt fine—no morning sickness, no fatigue. I was in peak form.

Until the spotting began.

I was in the ladies room at work and had just stripped down my underpants, settling onto the toilet seat with the blasé, automatic movement that we master in childhood. But blotches of red seeping into cotton and smearing toilet paper crashed into my awareness. Hot anxiety prickled up my arms and across my chest. I tried to think, to calm myself. Call the doctor. Get control. *You've got work to do!*

I always thought that miscarriages occurred quickly. I had seen the movies and television shows where the woman suddenly hunches over in pain, desperately grabbing the nearest chair for support before the quick cut to the hospital. Little did I know that a miscarriage could take days, even weeks—extended periods of time fraught with anxious uncertainty. I was forced to reveal to my boss that I was not only pregnant, but that I had to leave my desk piled with market analyses and manufacturing projections to follow doctor's orders and stay off my feet. As frosty January gales blew down New York City's streets, I sat in our flat, fearful of moving, and waited for my body to declare its decision.

About a week later, François came home one evening, sat on our bed and solemnly announced that his new boss had asked him to go on a business trip to China. China, the hot frontier of the early 1990s—1.2 billion people ripe for the invasion of Western products and services. I watched him, sitting there, struggling with reasons and obligations, helpless to stop whatever process had begun in my body. We discussed postponing the trip. We discussed the sympathetic, insincere response he would receive from his office, the potential impression he would make too early in a new job of being encumbered and unwilling to rise to every challenge. He left for China a few days later.

I would venture out, slowly and carefully over brittle mounds of snow, to the doctor's office for sonograms that showed dark masses of blood in my uterus and blood tests that measured abnormally low hormone increases. But the baby developed a heartbeat nonetheless and I felt hope, as well as a surge of maternal pride.

I didn't abandon that hope until the cramps came. I had been spotting for three weeks, but now blood trickled in bright, fresh streams down my legs. I called my doctor who gave me an address for a mid-town clinic. Contractions, deeper and stronger than I ever imagined for a miscarriage, clenched my abdomen in muscular strangleholds while I hailed a cab and sat in the clinic's waiting room. When the receptionist called me, she asked if I wanted to pay with cash or credit card. I pulled my wallet out of my back pocket, vaguely aware that my jeans were pasted to my inner thighs with blood, and handed her my Visa.

My doctor, a no-nonsense woman with the greyish pallor of fatigue, her hair escaping from a roughly-tied ponytail, whisked me into a room and deftly scraped away the remnants of my pregnancy. 'You'll feel crampy for awhile,' she declared as I stirred awake. And it was over. Gone.

In the following weeks, people told me that miscarriages happen to millions of women. But none of them were among the women in my life—not yet. Their range of perspectives was surprisingly broad. Some saw only a foetus, a mass of cells. Others told me it was all for the best—there was probably something wrong with it anyway. But, rightly or wrongly, rationally or irrationally, that cell group had become a fully-formed baby in my heart and mind, a child with warm breath and a soft, snug little body. Millions of women, yet I felt so alone with my grief.

I threw myself back into work. My boss had called me every day while I was gone to discuss business and check my progress. Initially he was genuinely sympathetic, but by the second week of my absence, irritation crept into his voice. He was being forced to manage tasks that were beneath him. So I worked late into the evening and over weekends to make up for lost time.

Looking back, I should have found a support group. I should have searched out four or five of those millions of women. For François, our miscarriage was a hiccup, a minor setback to put behind us. But I felt surrounded by reminders. As I dressed in the morning, I confronted a new fullness in my body. I continued to bleed for another two weeks. Around me, the number of babies and pregnant women seemed to multiply. They were in the streets, the supermarket, the video store—each of them creating an inescapable realisation that I'd had a child within me who had slipped away.

Through these ruminations, implications of my family history began weighing on me. Although my mother had carried children easily, my paternal grandmother was one of three sisters but the only one who had successfully carried a child to term. She had several miscarriages, a sombre footnote to her otherwise cheerful existence. One of her sisters had miscarried as well. There I was, blundering through melancholy after just one loss. The magnitude of heartbreak from another, from any more, would be nearly unbearable. Increasingly, I needed to understand *why* my miscarriage happened, to be assured that it wasn't due to an inherent weakness in me that risked repeating.

I called the lab that had studied the foetus. Except for revealing it had been a boy, they had no answers.

Having shown my intention to start a family, I wasn't surprised when I was shifted to a less demanding brand. Within six months I fell pregnant again. Within eight weeks I was bleeding.

Again, I went home and stayed there for nearly a month. I anticipated the worst, fretting over every abdominal twinge and examining my underwear each time I went to the bathroom. In my determination to understand why I kept bleeding, I switched to a specialist who diagnosed me with the helpless tendency for 'high risk' pregnancies, cause unknown. But this pregnancy held past twelve weeks and I returned to work cautiously. I continued to spot, went home whenever the brownish-red stains appeared, and counted the days into the twenty-six week threshold when chances grew that my baby would live if the pregnancy went awry. And when my daughter Nathalie was born in the middle of a March snowstorm, I pressed her to my chest with gratitude. She had made it and never had to depend on the instability of my womb again.

But another pregnancy would. I knew it. As I returned to work, leaving home at six-thirty am for the office and then coming back twelve hours later to mother into the night, I knew that my schedule combined with my faulty child-bearing would sabotage our attempt to grow our family further. Eventually I would have to make a choice: continue on my current career path and minimise our chances for a baby, or abandon it to maximise them.

Just a year later, I was forced to confront that decision. François was offered a transfer to Hong Kong—a promotion, good money, an opportunity he deserved. But I balked. I had been promoted myself, had finally regained my professional footing. If I agreed to go, I probably wouldn't land the same calibre of work in Hong Kong—the hurdles of visa attainment, childcare, commuting and job availability would be too great. I wasn't ready to decide, and I didn't want to.

On the morning train into New York City, François slipped his hand into mine and stated the truth that I had been avoiding. 'You wouldn't have to work,' he said gently. 'We could try to have another baby.'

Staring out the window at passing houses building into New York City's urban sprawl, I realised that somewhere along the trail of blood and cramps and the final, triumphant gasp of labour I had already made my choice. Nearly twenty years after my decision never to become a stay-at-home mother, the uncontrollable reality of motherhood had led me to become exactly that.

We moved to Hong Kong. Amidst the bustling fusion of steel-bright streets and decrepit laneways swathed in the ancient richness of south Chinese culture, I released myself to a life I never anticipated. Within four months, I was pregnant again. Nine weeks on, while walking up stairs I felt a light snap in the base of my abdomen, like the gentle click of fingers. Blood—more than I had experienced with my other pregnancies—soaked my shorts. I called François home, returned to the caged stillness of my bed, and braced for another end.

I made it through the night with light aches and twinges. The next day, I began the drill of filing off to the doctor's office for the sonograms and blood tests that I knew so well. But rather than taxiing through New York, I ferried from our home through Victoria Harbour where tugboats puttered between looming cargo ships and sampans glided over the water with slow, dignified grace.

Although my tests were normal, I continued to spot. Again, I was ordered to rest. I hired a live-in sitter—a young Philippine woman named May-May—to help look after Nat. At twenty weeks, too early to hope for a healthy delivery, I started having contractions. My doctor, a confident Englishman who moonlighted as a rugby umpire, prescribed tablets that quelled them. When the contractions started again, I called him in panic. 'Keep taking the tablets,' he soothed. 'Don't worry. I have patients who pop them like Smarties.'

Alone for hours, I was consumed with the awareness of my threatened pregnancy. But my belly grew with a life that heaved and kicked with increasing strength. After returning home from the park or a play date with her beloved May-May, Nat would run upstairs, fly onto my bed and press her head to my tummy. She had long since abandoned any hope that I would venture out with her. Instead, she seemed content to perceive me as a hen dutifully resting on her nest readying her chick to hatch.

At thirty-seven weeks, I gave birth to a son, Etienne. While François and my rugby umpire doctor cheered me on, my Christmas baby ploughed through me before the anaesthesiologist arrived from a holiday party. But I didn't mind. Far from it. He was worth every lonely hour, every day of worry, every moment of writhing labour.

But I would never try to fall pregnant again. I had gambled enough.

After four years in Hong Kong, François was transferred to France. There, I considered returning to work, but the complications and expense of childcare and commuting remained disincentives. The truth was, I preferred to be my children's home base as they confronted their international adventures—adventures that became part and parcel of my own. Finding and setting up a house within a small village in the Paris suburbs, establishing my kids in the local public school, and learning to cope with teachers, bank tellers, doctors, police and even the electrician within the French system, and all in French, imbued my domestic responsibilities with a particularly challenging edge. It was a lifestyle that forced me to be resourceful, take initiative and develop greater awareness of other people, places and cultures. Although it was not the path my younger self had envisioned, it was no less worthwhile—a bittersweet detour I would not have pursued if I had been able to carry children with normal ease.

Of course there were periods when I felt buried and belittled, recognised as my husband's wife and children's mother and not much more. When a sense of inadequacy hounded me for being a stay-at-home mum instead of the working mother I was psychologically groomed to become. Periods when our single-income dependence on a corporate world rife with acquisitions and bankruptcies made us terrifyingly vulnerable. It was during one such period that we decided to move to Australia. After three intercontinental moves in eight years, François and I were ready to plant roots, to call a special place home. That was nearly ten years ago.

I often think about that thirteen-year-old girl I once was. When I remember my decision to derail her dreams, I still sense her determination. But she's easier to soothe now, understanding that dreams can buffet and transform along a course that is as different, yet enriching, as anything she could imagine.

Christine Darcas has published both fiction and nonfiction in Australia and overseas. In Australia, her work has appeared in newspapers and magazines including Sunday Life *magazine,* Reader's Digest *and* Melbourne's Child. *She is the author of two novels published by Hachette Australia,* Dancing Backwards in High Heels *and* Spinning Out. *Christine lives in Melbourne with her husband and two teenage children.*

This Path Before

Tiffany Tregenza

It's my third, I think,
as I stare at the bright red pool of blood.
It's my third miscarriage.
I know,
without a single doubt in my mind,
that it is happening again.
I'm not sure how I feel.
Sad.
Numb.
Resigned.
There's a knock on the door.
Am I okay?
No.
'Yes,' I reply,
and quickly clean myself up.

There will be no baby now.
'Are you bleeding?' he asks as I come from the bathroom
(he is dressed for work
and I am suddenly resentful).
I nod
and begin to cry.
Three sets of little-girl-eyes settle on me;
they look worried,
so I swipe at the big, useless tears
and tell them Mummy is all right
but I can already feel the heavy cramps beginning
and the heat
low in my belly.
Not all right.
Never all right.
He asks what I need from him
and for some reason
I tell him,
'Go to work.'
I see the secret relief on his face.
He wants to escape.
'I'll call you if I get into trouble.'
It seems so matter-of-fact
but this is my third loss
and we have been down this path before.
I am only ten weeks along.
He leaves and I dress my girls.
I hug them tight.

I take some pain relief
and sit with them while they play babies.
The morning is both fast and slow
as *my* baby,
my hopes and dreams
trickle away,
and soon it's time for morning nap.
Three hours have passed since I discovered the damp red spot
on the sheets,
glaring at me like an evil eye
or an open wound.
Once they are asleep
I suddenly need to shower—
to cleanse (rid) myself
of this terrible happening.
The hot water brings out the pain
and the tears
and there is a lot of blood.
Too much.
I know,
almost instinctively,
that I am in trouble.
I ring him,
the father of this never-to-be baby
and tell him to come,
tell him
I am not okay.
The cramping is coming in constant waves

as the baby tries to leave me
without success
and I feel sick
and hot
and cold
all at once.
He is an hour away.
I need to carry on,
get organised,
have the girls looked after,
because I know
I will need him to come with me,
I know
that I cannot do this on my own
no matter how many times
I have miscarried before.
I will have to go to the hospital
and although the doctors will be swift and look at me with kind, sad eyes
they will use words like 'products of conception'
and 'missed abortion'
which sting
and pull at my heart.
No matter how they play their cards
she will always be a baby to me.
I am almost certain I am (was)
carrying another daughter.
I know that once I am there

the baby I have come to love,
come to imagine,
will be nothing more than a memory,
a few scratchings of post-surgical handwriting
on a stark white page,
a quickly forgotten bad day by everyone else
but me.
For a few moments
I go with the pain,
hang on to it
as I long to hang onto this baby.
I wonder if I will try again
or if it is time to cut my losses.
I decide that it can't be over, this child-bearing time,
just as he comes through the door.
I know I will risk it
for another chance.

Tiffany Tregenza is a mother, wife, wrangler of small sausage dogs and keeper of the zoo. She enjoys writing, especially on her blog (www.mythreeringcircus.com), and has found she has a passion for photography. In a former life, she was a midwife but is currently trying her hand at being a stay-at-home mum to several teenagers and five-year-old twins. She is addicted to ice-cream.

For Tristan: A Meditation on Loss, Grief and Healing

Nicole Breit

On Mother's Day, when I was nearly six weeks pregnant, I began to lose my baby.

The day before I'd spent time in the garden while my partner and our toddler napped. I was in the habit of talking to the baby in quiet moments—as I lay in bed in the morning, as I fell asleep at night, and that afternoon as I dug out weeds. I told my baby about our garden and imagined enjoying it with him next spring. I pictured him sleeping peacefully next to me in his basket while I passed the hours happily with my hands in the cool soil.

The next evening there was some spotting before bed, and by morning it had turned to heavier bleeding. I went to work, but over the course of the day felt ill with what seemed like food poisoning. I called my midwife who reassured me, and went to bed early. I lay awake all night, using a heat pad to soothe the cramps, and getting up to use the toilet over and over again.

At the hospital the next day the doctor performed a pelvic exam to check if my cervix was open. To my great relief, it wasn't. There was a fifty per cent chance the baby was fine. I slept more peacefully that night, unwilling to give up hope.

But in the morning the ultrasound technician seemed to take a long time to find my baby. After several minutes she left the room to fetch a doctor. I sat up and tried to see the image frozen on the ultrasound screen. I thought I recognised what must be my baby, and felt calm, ready to hear that everything was fine. The doctor came in, sat down, and glanced briefly at the screen. He told me that at this stage there should be a yolk sac. He was sorry, but there was nothing there.

In retrospect, a part of me already knew the pregnancy had ended. As I lay awake the night before the ultrasound I talked to the baby, gently repeating my words like a chant. *If you can't stay, I understand. I still love you, and I want to be your mummy very much. I hope you can find a way to be with me again. Goodbye little one.*

The days that followed felt long, like time had slowed down. I was still extremely ill and stayed in bed for hours. Trying to get over my illness and cope with the unexpected and devastating loss took most of my energy. Each day and night I wept, but especially at night. I spent hours visiting websites related to miscarriage. I found several sites that sold personalised memorial jewellery. When I saw the image of a handmade charm with a garnet bead, my heart felt newly pierced with grief. Garnet was the birthstone for a baby who, like mine, would have been born in January. I sobbed uncontrollably once more.

From experience, I knew that there were no shortcuts through grief. It is something you must simply move through, whether you have lost someone you have known your whole life or a baby you will never know. It is a dark tunnel of uncertain length. Reaching the end, you discover that initially inconceivable place where you can laugh without the terrible, guilty thought that you have somehow, for a moment, forgotten the life that is no more.

Some describe a miscarriage as an invisible loss because people generally aren't comfortable discussing it. But I knew that being left alone with my sorrow would compound it. I felt compelled to talk about it, to tell the story repeatedly in order to try and understand what had happened. I was determined that my baby's short time with me would be known.

The feelings I experienced in the weeks that followed my miscarriage were intense. I felt profoundly distrustful of my body. I had been through nine rounds of fertility treatment, and couldn't believe that my body would fail me in this way. I was angry that I couldn't make my body do what it was supposed to—protect and nurture my baby.

At the same time, I felt an internal disconnection. The loss had split me in two. I had returned to work, and to those around me I appeared to be recovering well. But every minute of the day I was excruciatingly aware of the truth—the real me was paralysed by overwhelming confusion and sadness. The 'me' that looked fine on the outside was far from fine in reality.

Inside I was seething with emotion. I was sad, but I also felt personally rejected. I was angry at myself and the baby. I even felt hateful toward the spirit that would accept my invitation to life, only to throw it back at me. I wondered what I had done to ruin my chance at motherhood, and retraced my steps over and over again to try and identify my fatal error. I had tried so hard, repeatedly, to have a successful pregnancy. I was frustrated by my lack of control, and by how easily other women could do what was impossible for me. Mostly, I ached terribly for the baby I wanted so badly, but who didn't want me.

I went to counselling to learn how to navigate my complex feelings, and find my way to the end of the tunnel. I began to search for information on how other women learned to heal from their miscarriages. I sought out creative expressions, but had difficulty finding texts and imagery that were not medical. The few I did find included Frida Kahlo's painting, *Henry Ford Hospital (Miscarriage in Detroit)*, Rachel Barenblat's series of poems, *Through*, and Tori Amos' album of songs written following a miscarriage, *From the Choirgirl Hotel*.

Each of these expressions was so genuine, so heartfelt, that they moved me and nudged me further along emotionally. But they were not enough to help me purge the deepest, darkest feelings I needed to loosen and let go. I needed to find my own way to express my grief. So I created a series of self-portraits, taking photos of my naked face and body. I drew a large 'X' in red lipstick across my empty belly and took a picture of that, too.

My counsellor encouraged me to do things to acknowledge my grief and honour the child I had lost. We gave the baby our favourite boy's name, Tristan. We each wrote him a letter. We made a memorial stone for our garden, the place where I last felt deeply connected to him. And as time went on, I slowly began to feel my two selves reintegrate. When the outer 'me' began to accurately reflect what was going on inside the true 'me', I knew the hardest part of the grief was behind me.

In her essay 'Intimate Strangers', Eve Joseph, a former hospice worker, writes that metaphor is the language of the dying. When a person is near death, it is not uncommon to hear them speak of a taxi waiting outside, or of driving a vehicle with failed brakes. As I grieved my miscarriage, my subconscious also seemed to grapple with the death of my baby in metaphor.

For months I had nightmares about burying a body in my backyard. I knew I wasn't responsible for the death, but I was always responsible for the burial. I had to keep the body a secret to avoid trouble from the authorities. I could never forget, no matter what happened next, that there was a dead body in my backyard. The night I confessed to my partner that I thought the dream might somehow be about our lost little boy—the theme of death, the burial in the backyard, the fear of shame, and need for secrecy—the nightmares ceased.

While metaphor may be the language of the dying (and of those coping with death), symbolism is the language of those grieving a miscarriage. Many parents refer to their lost babies as angels, and use angel imagery in their tributes and memorials. Symbolism is the perfect shorthand to represent something that has no form, something too elusive to capture. Something that was hidden and mysterious while it lived, and now is simply gone.

I needed symbols. There was no proof that my baby ever existed except for the blood test results filed at the lab. He died ten days before his first scheduled ultrasound. All I had was the memory of the phone call confirming my pregnancy, four entries in a pregnancy journal that would have held many more, and a few pictures of myself while pregnant. The small space of time when Tristan was with me felt dream-like, unreal.

For lack of ever being able to know, see, smell, touch, or cuddle my baby, to never know the colour of his hair, his smile or laugh, I was able to find him in unexpected places. My baby was there in the blood red bead of a pendant. He was in a garden sculpture of a fairy boy, eyes downcast, sitting with his face cupped in his hands. And he was there in the garden stone my partner and I made together.

At my last counselling session, I talked about wanting to try and get pregnant again. My fertility specialist said there was no reason to wait, and I could proceed next cycle if I wanted to. While I knew that I couldn't keep trying to have a baby indefinitely, I was willing to try one more time. I felt it might be what I needed to help me reach the end of the tunnel, but I also knew if the attempt was unsuccessful, it would be more devastating than ever.

Five weeks after my miscarriage, a new cycle began. I called the clinic and picked up my kit of needles, sterile water and drugs. The next week I went into the clinic for my usual monitoring, and on the first day of summer, left work early for my final IUI (intrauterine insemination). Two weeks later I was pregnant.

While I was thrilled and hopeful, I also felt reluctant to celebrate. This feeling continued throughout the first trimester, and I didn't truly enjoy the pregnancy until I was safely halfway through. By the end of my pregnancy I anticipated the birth, but didn't feel as connected to this baby as I had to the previous one. Throughout the pregnancy, I never spoke to him the way I'd constantly spoken to the one who couldn't stay.

My son was born in March. The moment he arrived, I held him close and didn't move. I didn't want to let him go. I didn't even look at his face. And I didn't know his gender until my midwife asked at the ten-minute point if my partner and I were curious. I could have waited longer to find out—boy or girl, it didn't matter to me. I was elated that I'd finally been able to bring my baby into the world. Nothing else mattered. After so much struggle, so much pain, so much loss, he was finally here.

While I instantly fell in love with my son, I never expected that he would compensate for the absence of my other baby, or make that absence less painful. I have not forgotten Tristan, and never will.

Nicole Breit lives in Vancouver, Canada with her partner and their two young children. She graduated with a Bachelor of Arts in English Literature from the University of Victoria and holds a Bachelor of Education from the University of British Columbia. She writes poetry as well as creative nonfiction, and her blog, Writing for My Life, can be found at www.nicolebreit23.blogspot.com

On Reflection
Christine O'Neil

There it was again, the question I dreaded. Such an innocent question, but one that always made me catch my breath. A question I should be used to answering, but wasn't.

At social gatherings, school events or whenever a group of women who didn't know each other got together, the safest conversation was children.

'How many kids have you got, Chris?'

When I answered six, there was always the inevitable gasp and raised eyebrows. This was usually followed by, 'You must be very fertile,' or 'I can't imagine being pregnant six times'.

I would smile and nod and want to add, *In truth I've been pregnant eleven times*, but I never did. I knew this would lead to more questions. I was fortunate to produce six healthy babies—especially as I had the last four later in life, beginning when I was thirty-nine and ending when I was forty-six—but in between my babies were five miscarriages, and I remember each one.

I married young and, always idealistic, I told anyone who would listen that I wanted six children. Two miscarriages and two children later, my first marriage fell through and the prospect of any more children seemed to have faded.

But eight years later I married again. My second husband was eleven years younger than me and was keen to start a family. At this stage I was thirty-seven and we had no idea if my 'plumbing' still worked. Happily, not long after the wedding I was pregnant. We were thrilled, and my two eldest children were delighted that they would soon have a baby to play with.

Our joy was short-lived and, as was my pattern, I reached twelve weeks and began to spot. Tiny drops of dark brown blood that went on for days. 'Just rest and try not to worry and nature will take its course,' was the message from the medical world. I hated nature.

Platitudes from well-meaning family and friends—'If it's meant to be, the baby will be all right'—made me to want to yell, *Of course it's meant to be, I'm pregnant, aren't I?*

I lost that baby. My feeling of failure was awful. I had lost our first baby but my new husband said very little about what *he* felt and kept telling me that he was sure everything would be fine. He was certain we would have our family. All I wanted to do was curl up and think about the tiny life I had lost, the life my body had expelled. But there was no chance of that. I had two school-age children to care for and a job to go back to.

Not long after, I conceived again and edged gingerly past the dreaded twelve-week mark. A few weeks later I began to breathe again. I enjoyed the rest of the pregnancy and delivered a healthy baby girl.

With two teenagers and a toddler we needed more room. We decided to buy a block of land and build our dream home. There is a saying, 'New house, new baby,' and when we moved into our new house I was pregnant with our second baby.

At four weeks pregnant I felt like Mother Earth. We spent the weekends attempting to turn our sandy patch of dirt into a child-friendly garden. On one particular trip to the nursery to buy plants I saw a tiny Lilly Pilly tree. Its botanical name, *Acmena*, means 'bountiful', and indeed I felt very bountiful that day with a new life inside my womb. For some reason these trees felt symbolic to me, so we bought two and later that afternoon found them a new home in our back garden.

Four weeks became eight with no problems and eight became twelve. Once more I began to feel uneasy. I tried to stay calm. My breasts were swollen so I reasoned that this was a good sign. I felt a little nauseous in the evenings so that must be good too—clearly I had hormones supporting this pregnancy. I didn't drink coffee or alcohol and tried to rest. I say *tried*, as working part-time and chasing after three kids when I was at home left little time for resting.

Thirteen weeks dawned and I breathed a sigh of relief. This pregnancy was going well, or so I thought. One morning not long after my husband left for work, I became aware of a dull ache in my pelvic area followed by a damp feeling between my legs. A hasty trip to the bathroom confirmed my suspicions when a small amount of bright fresh blood trickled from me.

I sat there stunned. Not again, please God not again. It had all been going so well, I had done everything right. My diet had been textbook perfect, there wasn't a beneficial vitamin, mineral or enzyme I hadn't consumed. I went for gentle walks every day to keep fit. I wasn't overweight and my blood pressure was normal. This all seemed so unfair, so hard to understand. *Why me?* There was no answer.

'Mum, we're going,' called my thirteen-year-old daughter about to leave for school with her brother.

'Hang on,' I replied and walked slowly back to the kitchen. My daughter is now thirty-seven and still remembers that morning well. I kissed them goodbye, told them to go carefully on their bikes and issued the usual, 'Have a good day.'

She recalls standing by the front door, school bag in hand, watching me pick up the phone to call my husband. I reached for it with my right hand and, becoming aware of a wet feeling, I placed my left hand under my nightie and caught something. I will never forget looking down at the palm of my hand and seeing a circle of blood. There in its centre lay my baby, silvery pink and curled like an unfurled frond of fern.

For weeks afterwards I felt let down by my body, by God and by life itself. I tried not to let my grief affect my family. Often after my husband went to work and the big kids went to school, I would take my toddler daughter outside and we would sit beside the Lilly Pilly trees. She would play and I would cry. Was it something I'd done or something I hadn't? I scoured medical books for the cause, but they merely stated that between ten and twenty per cent of all pregnancies end in miscarriage. Cold comfort. I wanted reasons not generalisations. It was hard to face, but maybe I was too old.

On reflection, what kept me going was the inner belief that I would have my six children. Deep inside I knew that somehow I could do it. Finding the right doctor was very important and if I felt the doctor and I weren't on the same wavelength then I sought another who was. I read everything I could get my hands on. I asked questions (I'm sure my medical files were labelled, 'Inquisitive,' or less politely, 'Difficult patient!') and even though I couldn't find the reason for my miscarriages, I felt as if I was doing something positive that might influence the outcome of future pregnancies. Having a supportive partner helped me in my darkest moments, of which there were a few. His love and understanding kept me going.

Now, at sixty-two, I can report that my next pregnancy was trouble-free and at forty-one I gave birth to a baby girl. This was followed by one more miscarriage and two more healthy babies. I have been blessed. I got my six children, but I will never forget those five babies that didn't make it.

As for the Lilly Pilly trees, we sold the house and moved interstate many years ago. Recently, I visited our old home and was saddened to see that the trees had been removed. When I asked why, I was told they grew too big and their berries made too much mess. The owner asked if they were of any special significance to me. 'No,' I replied as the memories came flooding back. I lied.

Christine O'Neil loves to write. When not tending her veggie patch or working as a nurse, she can be found in her writing shed in the back garden. Mother of six and grandmother of two, she is midway through writing a historical and partly factual novel based in Perth, Western Australia.

Letting Go
Choe Brereton

The drum of his heartbeat echoed through the room, racing like a startled rabbit. Each brisk flub-dub rose and fell across the blinking screen. His miniature form was a nebulous lump that would soon differentiate into skin and muscle, bones and vital organs. I laughed from relief, not really aware until now how much I dreaded the sight of another vacuous space. During the last pregnancy a little over three months ago the first scan was inconclusive, the second, two weeks later, confirmed our fears. She had barely matured past a wad of cells, yet had awakened that same viscous love we now felt for the shapeless bean on the screen.

    At close to three months, Lump, as he affectionately became known, had already rolled my belly out a little way. My jeans still fastened at the waist but I felt chunky in them. I was sick, barely able to brush my teeth without throwing up, and at some point my nose had been swapped for that of a bloodhound's. The pantry was the worst. Extra virgin olive oil, even with the cap screwed tightly, made my stomach clutch—as did the sight of ginger hair. But for a time at least, I relished the frequent 'green' dashes, taking my discomfort to be a sign of his healthy growth.

My husband took to treating him like a gurgling newborn, asking him questions he couldn't possibly answer and kissing him frequently through the wall of my stomach. And until we knew otherwise, Lump remained a boy. We fantasised about his personality (easygoing), and his looks (amber eyes and caramel skin). By three months I had grown increasingly protective of him, sometimes overly so, like a ruffled and bawling goose.

And then one morning I saw the blood.

Dark sinuous veins that dolloped onto the shower floor and disappeared in gummy threads down the plughole. I must have cried out because my husband was suddenly at the shower door, eyes on the bloodied tiles, then on me, like I was some sort of apparition. I swabbed away tears with the heel of my hand; he reached through with a towel. 'We need to get to the hospital,' he said evenly, arms suddenly around me.

At our wardrobes we scrabbled through our things. I stretched on a pair of jeans, threw make-up in a bag. Deodorant hissed into the air. Down the hall the garage door clattered open as the remote put out its silent command. And then we were both in the car, looking a little like we had dressed in the dark. At my feet lay my cluttered handbag and films from previous scans—proof that life *did* pulse away in me.

We drove the familiar route, down country roads that meandered like agitated serpents. Horses in paddocks blurred past; cows were there, then gone. And all the while I thought of nothing else but what our baby was going through. He couldn't possibly understand what was happening, why his heart suddenly failed to beat properly—or at all.

I held my stomach the entire way as if trying to keep him from falling out, but by the time we arrived at the Early Pregnancy Unit I had shed most of my placenta. The doctor saw us quickly and the nurse tried to be reassuring, but their diligent examination turned up nothing more than another dark and empty space on the ultrasound. The screen was angled away, but I watched as one by one their shoulders slackened. Our baby, fully developed at twelve weeks and alive by every definition, was suddenly gone. This time I did not hinder the pain that threatened to split me in two. My husband pulled me close and wept into my ribs. The doctor ordered tests. The nurse, as gentle as my own mother, gave me a hug.

It was over a week later before I could face the thought of holding a service. It would be nothing big, just the two of us and a balloon to release once it was over. In the dimming light of a balmy October evening we inscribed on a heart-shaped balloon a simple but sincere message: *Our dearest Hope, we love you. Mum and Dad.*

We sat in the gloom, a candle lit before us, and prayed for him. And at the pinnacle of sunset, against the backdrop of a fiery sky, we stood on the balcony and let the gathering winds carry his balloon away. It wriggled through the branches of a nearby tree then shrank away to a dot before disappearing out of sight.

He was the second child we had lost in six months and by far the hardest one to let go of. From the moment we heard his heartbeat we were in love. In the end we named him Hope, because despite never holding him he had given us plenty. To think of him still makes our eyes sting, but we are assured that there will be a next time—and there will be.

Choe Brereton has had a varied and interesting writing career. Her work has appeared in a number of publications, both print and online, including Cosmos, The Helix, Alive *and* WHITE. *When she is not furiously working to meet a deadline, she enjoys reading children's literature and spending time with her very charming husband.*

The Visitor
Sally O'Brien

For all my certainty about my first pregnancy something was missing, and it turned out to be time. I had barely any of it before I miscarried. The brevity of my pregnancy sometimes made me question if I was even entitled to grieve.

We'd tried to get pregnant to see 'if everything still worked', and it happened with disconcerting ease, but because of our age and because it was still early days, we kept it quiet. When I found myself staring at two little stripes on a stick I felt quietly, tentatively happy, but not able to shout from the rooftops. Only he and I knew.

At times I suspected that our lack of declared intention to others to start a family somehow played a part in what happened, even though I knew this wasn't rational. The necessity of cloaking my pregnancy came to create the niggling thought that subterfuge had made the baby feel unwelcome and forced it to go elsewhere. In my mind, the act of keeping mum (oh, the irony) became inexorably tangled up with the loss itself.

Seven weeks pregnant and approaching Christmas, we flew from where we live in Switzerland to Australia, where I'm from, and I made an appointment with a doctor to discuss the pregnancy. She asked if I was sure I was pregnant and I told her that my cycle was so regular I could be certain. That and the double-striped stick, although not having it as proof made me feel as if I had come unprepared. I didn't want her to see me as some woman in her late thirties afflicted with a severe case of wishful thinking. I didn't tell her that her questions, and my unscientific-sounding responses, gave me pause, despite my certainty. By her calculations our baby would be born on 11 August. I know a lot of people born around that time of year, and it pleased me to think that I would be adding my baby's birthday to the mix.

We spent the next few days catching up with friends, often in a celebratory mood thanks to the season, but we didn't share our news. We decided to wait until we passed the first trimester mark. I ordered decaffeinated coffee and nursed glasses of wine, pretending to sip in order to avoid the inevitable 'Are you pregnant?' queries.

Later that week we were at the accountant's getting my tax done. She asked if we had kids. My husband and I looked at each other with a smile and the accountant became the first person to know and offer us congratulations. And, as it turned out, the last.

Only minutes later I experienced mild cramping in my abdomen. I assumed it was something normal associated with pregnancy, although I was disconcerted by how much the cramps resembled period pain. And I had started bleeding. I said nothing though, too rattled to give voice to my suspicion that something was wrong.

Some fifteen minutes later I called the GP from our car and left a message. We drove to a friend's house nearby and I asked if she had a sanitary pad. She looked at me strangely, no doubt wondering why I'd come all the way to her place to drop in and ask for such a thing. So I told her what was going on and she became the second person to know, although I already suspected that it was too late, and that I was no longer pregnant.

We got back into the car and the doctor phoned. She told me it might indeed be spotting, or it might be a miscarriage and that I needed to look for foetal tissue. Her lack of a definitive answer made me feel even less certain of things, and I began to cry. In the emotion of the moment I felt as though nothing about being pregnant had been certain, not even my miscarriage, which started in an accountant's office and was being discussed over the phone as I sat in a car in a bayside Melbourne suburb. My friend, seeing that we were still parked outside her house, came out with her melancholy-eyed greyhound and hugged us some more.

That night, I sat on a friend's couch far from home, blanketed and numbed, eating take-away laksa with a cold beer, watching the news. The cramps were a dull pain muted by painkillers. It was over.

The next morning was the hardest. Waking up in a bed that wasn't mine in a house that wasn't my home and realising that only yesterday, at this exact time in the morning, I had been pregnant. And now I wasn't. Every day that followed would take me a little further away from the time I had been pregnant. I didn't have any blood tests results, or photographs of a tiny form with a heartbeat to prove what I had held inside. I knew I was pregnant. And then I knew I wasn't. What I didn't know was if I would ever get pregnant again. Maybe this was my one shot at being a mum.

It was the season when people reveal their plans for the coming year, and even though everyone I spoke to in the days after my miscarriage was a good friend, I never felt that I could tell them that only recently I had been a mother-to-be. That I had been planning to spend the new year preparing to have a baby. Plans I hadn't even given proper shape to were derailed. What stretched before me now was uncertainty and a grief that kept getting put on the backburner amidst the seasonal celebrations.

We had a long drive to my hometown of Sydney ahead of us, and I welcomed the space and time it would give me to think about what had happened. Yet after so much avoidance the idea also left me wary. During the hours between the two cities my husband and I sat side-by-side, saying little but glad to be near the one person who knew what the other was thinking.

The fact that I had been carrying life and now wasn't left me hollow. My earlier bravado in telling myself and my husband that we would enjoy life whether we had children or not lacked conviction. Something—*someone*—was missing, and to add to the sadness, I felt that I had not properly appreciated being pregnant. I found myself in a foreign state—this place called Loss. Even though I knew there were countless other people who had been there I felt isolated. I could find no map for such territory. It was a different loss to others I had experienced, where lovers, friends and even family had gone from my life. I had lost someone I didn't yet know.

One of the oddest things about my miscarriage was that I felt sheepish about it. As though it was my fault and I should have been able to prevent it. At times, I am still reluctant to talk about it because I compare my early loss with other more tragic stories. What happened to me doesn't really count when compared with the grief and loss of women who were further along in their pregnancies and had 'more to lose'. It was as though my miscarriage was the result of some foolishness, something to be embarrassed about.

We returned home to Europe in full winter. I never bothered to call the doctor in Melbourne again. There had been no problems with my miscarriage as far as I could tell—only the fact of the miscarriage itself. I fell ill with bronchitis and had some poor blood test results and reluctantly told a Swiss doctor about what had happened. I didn't want to be questioned about whether I'd had a proper examination during or after, about whether I'd really been pregnant. My doctor was sympathetic and made it clear that I needed to rest and let my body return to health.

In the months that followed I grew stronger until I felt ready to get pregnant again. I counted days in the hope that if I paid enough attention, if I was *mindful* this time, I would fall pregnant and stay that way for the whole nine months. Yet it was hard to ignore that falling pregnant was a hit-and-miss affair. There were no guarantees and often no logic to it. People who wanted children sometimes remained childless, others fell pregnant by accident.

By early May, I knew I was pregnant again, and this time I was certain of what I felt. Cautious but profoundly grateful. I was stronger and surer. Even so, for several nights in a row during my second trimester I was unable to sleep. During one of these nights I lay on the couch in darkness, eyes watering and nose running uncontrollably, wondering what on earth I could possibly be reacting to. Just as dawn lightened the living room walls, I realised. This was when my other baby had been due. It was 11 August. I had put the date to the back of my mind, but something had brought me back to grieve. Even if my mind had failed to join the dots on my calendar, my body had known and taken the time to mourn again. My body literally woke me up to what I had tried to ignore.

Despite this episode of renewed grief, my pregnancy continued smoothly. In the middle of winter our baby entered the world with a lusty cry. When he was placed on my chest we searched for each other, and I knew immediately that he was a part of me. But that other little baby—who went away far too soon and who I never got to know—was also part of me. At last, I was sure of my feelings.

Sally O'Brien is an Australian freelance writer and editor, based in Lausanne, Switzerland, where she lives in a cosy old apartment with her husband, photographer Denis Balibouse, and their toddler son. She writes short stories, nonfiction and never-ending lists while her child sleeps. She blogs at www.swissingaround.blogspot.com

Swords, Guns and Superheros
Becki Brown

My first pregnancy and the subsequent birth of my first child went so smoothly that I believed I was invincible. I had no real difficulty conceiving, although at the time I believed there might be an issue somehow related to the excess of dark hormonal hair that plagued me. In fact, the six months it took my body to be free of years of contraceptive pill use was quite normal. That first child slid into this world, into my own hands, attended by a midwife, his father and my parents. The obstetric gynaecologist (obgyn) that I'd been seeing for eleven months was just in time to sew up the damage and give me a pat on the back. I felt like some sort of maternity goddess. I was on top of the world. I was in control of all things.

Of course when you're that high up you must eventually come back down, and for me it happened with a fall. When we decided eighteen months later that it was time to add a daughter to the family I got pregnant very quickly. I contacted the same midwife who helped deliver my first child, believing that spending the money on an obgyn was not necessary. At the first visit, the midwife was concerned that I was already bigger than I should have been at eight weeks, and that perhaps I was having twins. An ultrasound scan a week later did reveal twin sacs, one more developed than the other with a beating heart. When I look back now, the sonographer was probably just being gentle when she told me it was too early to rule either way on the second sac, but I was convinced that I was having twins.

A week later I woke feeling feel sad and lethargic. The following day I started to bleed. An ultrasound was arranged. I lay on the bed staring at the little screen, amazed by the differences I could clearly see. The sac with the viable foetus had grown, showing the potential to one day look human, but it was still, without a heartbeat. Both our babies had died. All I could think was, *It must be a mistake.* Surely this wasn't happening to me.

They scheduled a curette for later in the week, but when I started to bleed more heavily they decided to keep me overnight and perform surgery early the next day. In a cruel twist, as there was no other place for me, I spent the night in the paediatric wing right next to the maternity ward. I had meant to go there again, but not like that.

Towards the end of the year I got pregnant again. It lasted eight weeks and disappeared without much fuss. I passed a one-centimetre twisted shell-shaped clot while waiting in the hospital for my baby's first ultrasound.

The ultrasound of pregnancy number four showed a heartbeat, polycystic ovaries, and a small fibroid growing on the side of my uterus. When the bleeding started I hoped against all odds that it was okay, but another baby had died inside me.

With each miscarriage I felt my sense of failure deepen. It became everything to me to have another full-term pregnancy. Another child. A girl. I was obsessed, and I felt completely alone. None of the baby books and magazines talked much about miscarriage, and my friends and family all shied away from an obviously painful subject. I couldn't accept that I wasn't meant to have any more children. I insisted on being referred to different doctors and specialists, believing that the polycystic ovaries and the excess hair must be the problem.

I lost pregnancy number five almost as soon as the pregnancy test confirmed its existence. Every month that my period came I felt that I had failed all over again.

My obgyn referred me to an endocrinologist (a hormone specialist). They both recommended taking a break from trying to have a baby. Then the endocrinologist also offered me an answer and possible treatment for the riddle of my excess hair, which apparently had nothing to do with my inability to have a baby. If that wasn't the reason, what was? My head was fizzing with confused thoughts and emotions. So I chose to take the time out and trial a hair reduction medication, requiring me to go on the pill and quit smoking again.

The next six months was a time of soul-searching and growth for me. I came to accept the way I looked, and realised that I needed to find faith in myself again. You are told that a miscarriage is not your fault—it is something to do with nature, blah blah blah. But you still blame yourself because it happens inside you. Nevertheless I realised that I wanted to keep trying. I was not ready to give up on that dream yet.

This time I got pregnant my first month off the pill. I felt back on top of the world, things were going to be just right. I had quit smoking, I would be careful what I ate and what I did. This was it. I had done some soul searching, cleaned up my act, and was now ready to get on with the business of having a child, any child.

I was standing in front of the hospital when I started smoking again. Six months of nicotine abstinence easily forgotten as I paced under the hospital verandah, emotionally preparing myself like a boxer before a big fight. I had discovered the bleeding first thing that morning. No pain, not at first, just a pinkish wipe on toilet paper. Because I had been through this heartbreakingly familiar scene so many times before, I knew deep down how it was going to end. Yet only a week before I had seen my baby on the ultrasound screen, a beautiful peanut shape with a beating heart. I needed another visual to see for myself what had changed.

The emergency waiting area was ugly, harsh and mostly grey—an apt reflection of my mood. I sat on the edge of my seat, feeling twists and turns in my abdomen and hoping they were caused by nerves, not a contracting uterus.

A male sonographer called my name. I had done this many times before. I knew what was coming. But I had never been examined by a man and I miserably added this discomfort to the overflowing bucket of emotions I was carrying.

I went through the routine of shedding my pants and knickers, climbing onto the examination bed and under the supplied blanket. When the transducer was placed on my stomach I held my breath. My husband and I stared at the screen. My eyes bored into its hazy surface, drawing a baby picture from my own wishes. But although spots swirled all over the screen I could see no peanut-shaped baby. Where did it go? The sonographer kept searching, although I'm sure it was just to mollify me.

'Are you sure you were even pregnant?' he asked patronisingly, as if I had not been so six times before.

I wanted to yell at him for being rude, for being a man, for finding nothing—but my energy was flowing out of me at an alarming rate. I could feel myself deflating.

'I saw this pregnancy last week,' I told him. 'The heart was beating …' I trailed off at the sceptical look on his face.

'Well I can see no evidence of it, but we'll conduct a transvaginal exam just to be sure. You should go and empty your bladder.'

I did as requested and felt my heart plummet when I wiped myself and felt something solid. I brought the toilet paper up to inspect it, my sanity cracking as I saw my tiny foetus, complete and still safe within its amniotic sac. It looked just like a picture from a textbook. Holding it in my shaking hands, I rested my head against the wall and cried.

But this was something. Surely there was some important scientific reason why my body had expelled a perfect-looking foetus. I nervously took my toilet paper-wrapped findings to the sonographer. *Here's your bloody proof*, I thought. Shock was setting in. I stumbled over my words, explaining to both the sonographer and my husband what had happened in the toilet, and held out my scientific package. The sonographer shrunk away from it, refusing to take it from me.

'Shouldn't I keep this?' I asked. 'Where should I put it? Surely somebody should be inspecting this?'

But he told me there was no use keeping it—I should go and flush it down the toilet. I was mortified and humiliated, but did as I was told. The rest of the examination was a blur. I could feel that my husband was completely lost on his own, but I was busy processing the outcome of this pregnancy with both mourning and wonder.

Back in the dismal waiting area I called my obgyn and brokenly told him everything. When he asked me what had happened to the foetus, I fell apart, crying that they'd told me to flush it. He actually swore! I wanted to, but he did. Then he told me that he had some new ideas, to come and see him next week. I left the hospital deflated but slowly filling with a new hope. I had miscarried in the hospital toilet, but my obgyn had a new plan.

Within the next month I met my obgyn again in the operating theatre. He smiled and crossed his fingers before the anaesthetist put me under and my obgyn (also a surgeon) sewed my cervix closed with a single stitch. It would allow sperm through, but not much else.

The theory went like this—since the birth of my first child my cervix had become less competent and my uterus irritable.

This meant that any small tremor in my uterus, like an orgasm, could set off a labour-like reaction where my cervix dilated and expelled the pregnancy. So my cervix was stitched up and when I got pregnant again I was given a script for medication to stop my uterus from contracting. I was banned from sex and, specifically, from having an orgasm.

Nine months later I gave birth to a healthy baby boy by emergency caesarean section. The fibroid, which had been considered harmless a few years ago, grew with the hormones to block the exit to my womb. My baby got stuck. It seemed as though nature was giving me a helping hand to keep him in there.

The six years between my first two children were like a theme park ride that travels up, up, up, peaks very high, and then comes down so hard and fast that it crashes. Somehow you survive and do it all over again, bits of you broken but still able to function.

My third son was also carried to term with the aid of a cervical stitch and delivered by planned caesarean section. During the surgery my tubes were tied, officially ending twelve years of trying to have babies. I may not have a daughter, but I am madly in love with my sword, gun, and superhero-loving family.

Becki Brown is currently studying a Bachelor of Arts in Literature at Griffith University. She lives on fifty acres with her rose-growing husband and three noisy boys. She loves to read and write fiction with a romantic or historical flavour.

A Perfect Square
Rosalind McKenzie

My head doesn't feel big enough. There isn't room for this thought. It only feels big enough to look out of the lounge room window and see the afternoon sun making lacework out of the trees and know that it is beautiful. But my head does not feel big enough to think about the steady flow of blood and the dull pain in my lower belly. When I try to think about that, it's as if my head has filled with thick liquid and there isn't room for a drop more.

Yours was a silent death. No one saw the moment that you died. But there must have been one, a moment when you were alive one second and not alive the next. I wonder what I was doing at that moment. Was I washing dishes? Was I driving to work? If I was thinking about you at all, it was about your life not your death.

They tell me that you were still alive three days ago. When I planted the front garden you were still with me. As I worked,

I imagined the garden through your eyes. I chose livid pink azaleas and a flamingo-tinted magnolia because I thought you would like bright colours.

Yours was a lonely death. Perhaps the most lonely of all. No one ever saw you or touched you. No one knew if you were male or female. No one knew if your eyes were brown or green. No one knew if you had curly hair like your father. You never understood what life was about and yet you were expected to die alone.

I wonder if you struggled. Did you kick or did you slip quietly into death, life ebbing away until the last spark was gone? They tell me that you couldn't feel pain but they don't know everything. They don't even know why you died.

I had an ultrasound today to confirm that you had gone. In the waiting area there were women who stroked their stomachs tenderly and smiled at their husbands. On the reception desk there was a little sign about paying five dollars for a video, pictures of the baby. But on my screen there was only black and white haze that the nurse called the 'products of conception'.

I went to the day clinic to arrange an operation for tomorrow. The woman at the desk made jokes about private health insurance and told me that she was having a bad day. I smiled when I was supposed to and answered her questions. There was a form to fill in and a box that I had to tick if I was pregnant. I left it blank, a small white perfect square.

Tomorrow morning I'll go back to the clinic. I'll sit in the waiting room among the polished pot plants and the *Vogue* magazines and listen to the television. Then they'll call my name and I'll follow their instructions and strip naked and put on a hospital gown and lie on a hospital trolley. They'll wheel me into the theatre and everyone will smile at me from behind their surgical masks and say that everything will be all right. But I will know that they are lying; everything will not be all right.

So, I sit here in the lounge room and gaze through the window into the back garden and try to concentrate on thoughts that can fit inside my brimming head. The jasmine vine needs to be tied back and the lattice work is loose. I notice that the mango tree is laden with flowers, but this is Sydney and it's too cold for it to bear any fruit.

You were small enough to fit into the palm of my hand and yet the void you left is large enough for me to drown in.

Rosalind McKenzie loves to paint, travel and write short stories. She is a Gifted Education Coordinator but also teaches Film and English at Newington College in Sydney. She has a husband, a son, five cats and a cavalier spaniel.

Sorrow Comes Unsent For
Lou Pollard

'I want a pink one, not a blue one. It's *my* birthday,' the six-year-old girl screamed. She glared up at me with fierce eyes as I felt a sharp spasm across my lower abdomen. I wiped my face on the frill of my costume and fumbled for a bright pink balloon. What was happening? I looked around at the parties full of children—the glare of the flashing disco lights, the crash of the pins, the squealing sounds of *I'm A Barbie Girl, in a Barbie World* blaring at full volume from the speakers.

It was late summer and I was dressed as a clown making balloon animals in a cavernous bowling alley when I was gripped by sudden intense stomach cramps. I remember thinking, *I have to make about twenty more balloon dogs, then I'll get the hell out of here.* By the time I reached my car, sweat trickled down my back and red make-up ran down my chin. I drove home without stopping, the Saturday afternoon market traffic a blur, as a stabbing sensation burned through my lower back. When I got home I thought, *Maybe I'm not pregnant, I'm bleeding. This period is really intense.*

Lying on my bed was agony, so I drove down the street to the emergency department of my local hospital. My husband stayed home with our baby daughter. I hobbled in to see the triage nurse and she told me to wait for a doctor. I tried to take a seat like a normal person, but the pain was so bad I couldn't sit down on the hard plastic chairs in the packed waiting room.

In between spasms I made my way to the ladies toilet. Holding onto the wall I rocked my hips like a deranged belly dancer and leaned over, my head almost in the tiny sink as I tried to cope with the tremors rocking my body. I pulled my pants down and sat down on the seat. And with one mighty contraction my nine-week-old foetus popped out and went down the S-bend. I stood up, my pants around my ankles. I meant to push the emergency aid button but instead I accidentally stepped on the flush pedal near the floor. I flushed my baby down the toilet.

'Why didn't you fish it out of the toilet? You shouldn't have flushed it, we needed to see it,' said the irate nurse on duty. I stared at her dumbstruck, I had no idea what I'd just done. It felt like one minute I was wearing a silly hat and the next I was bleeding in a hospital bathroom.

I was taken by ambulance to RPA Hospital by a lovely ambo who kept coming back to visit me throughout the night, after he delivered the drug addicts and drunks he picked up on the crazy Saturday night streets. While I waited for a bed at the maternity hospital across the road, I asked him why he wanted to be a paramedic.

'Don't the crack addicts get to you?' I said.

'I like to help people, I'm good at it. Where's your bloke?'

'I, ah, he's at home, with our daughter. He doesn't drive,' I said as my ambo friend rushed away again.

During the night my daughter was screaming so much my sister drove her to me at three am to be breastfed. At six am I was wheeled across the road to the hospital where I'd given birth to her nine months before. The building was so rundown that there was no hot water and the women's magazines were so old one issue had baby photos of Prince Charles in it. I stayed for a few hours on the ward but the sound of new babies crying was more than I could bear so my sister drove me home.

Two days later she took me back to the same hospital for a D and C. My mother came with us; my artist husband was too busy creating. As I breastfed my child in the crowded day surgery waiting room, two women looked at her with longing. I felt guilty and greedy. We were all waiting for the same procedure, but I already had a baby. These women obviously had none.

One of the doctors said my excessive intake of Vitamin A might have caused my miscarriage. Seven weeks before I was so tired when we returned from a 'holiday' at my mother-in-law's house that I took too many vitamin pills prescribed by an old friend of my husband's, Neil the amateur herbalist.

I remember trying to grab the hand of the anaesthetist before I went under. I wanted to say, 'Help me, I've lost my baby.'

But it was too late. A life had gone and none of the doctors could bring him back. *Him.* I had an overwhelming feeling that I'd lost a boy. As an orderly wheeled me into theatre I thought, 'I'll never have a son.'

When the faceless nurse placed the mask on my mouth I prayed I'd sleep for hours, but I woke up after twenty minutes and it was done. In the car afterwards my mother said, 'You'll have another one,' and I couldn't reply.

It wasn't until I was in my own bed that it hit me. I'd lost a child. My baby girl had lost a sibling. I buried my sadness—I was too tired and too busy with night feeds and nappy changing, mostly on my own, to deal with it. And my childless best friends wouldn't understand.

I woke up in the middle of the night a week later and thought, 'Why did I flush that toilet? I didn't even look at my baby.' If he had lived my daughter would now have a spotty thirteen-year-old brother. I had even picked a name for him.

Lou Pollard is a single mother of three daughters, comedian, actor, clown doctor and speaker. She was the literary assistant and collaborator on ten books with her father, Jack Pollard, one of Australia's most prolific writers. She has contributed to anthologies, written for Planet Ark and Essentially Me *e-magazine, and speaks to community and corporate groups for the Humour Foundation on how to relieve stress with laughter. She blogs at http://loupollard.wordpress.com*

Butterfly Nets
Tracey Slater

Unless we document everything at the moment it happens, we mostly forget what has gone before. Much of life consists of inconsequence and insignificance; time slipping away like mercury, fleeting moments captured with a pen or camera. But events of true import require no such thing. They are inescapably tangled in the butterfly nets of our memory.

It was my first miscarriage. Twelve weeks into my pregnancy I noticed that my breasts felt cushiony again, no longer the painful leaden balloons they had been in past weeks. I redeveloped a hankering for wine and coffee, instead of experiencing nausea at the mere mention of those words. Then the thin brown spots came. A midwife by profession, I knew a long-held dream was disintegrating.

An ultrasound confirmed my fears. My babies had died early on; there were two as it turned out. Barely visible pinpricks—my twins, my babies, my hopes—were suspended, lost and non-living, each in its own robust, comparatively gigantic bag of membranes.

'As you can see here, these embryos haven't formed beyond a couple of weeks, you have to strain to see them,' said the doctor. 'Blighted ovum we call it, blighted ova in your case. This pregnancy cannot progress. I'm so very sorry.'

Cut to afterwards, following the operation that concluded the physical aspect of my trial. A nurse told me, kindly but firmly, that I had to eat, drink and pass urine 'without ill effects' before I could leave the hospital. I nodded obediently, sipped some water and half-heartedly swallowed some unappetising blancmange. But mostly I wept, bothering a growing mound of sodden paper tissues that I shredded to pulp between my fingers.

Then she came—a middle-aged, brittle-haired blonde. She introduced herself and pulled up a chair which was spilling stuffing through a tear in the vinyl. She looked at me directly with grey-blue eyes whose turned-down corners suggested that over time she had become weighed down by other people's tragedies.

She told me how sorry she was and asked me a few questions, including how I was feeling and whether I could rely on good emotional support at home. I answered with the seal-like sounds I normally make when my emotional banks have burst. She didn't have to ask how I was feeling. Not really. She nodded. My incoherence must have made sense somehow.

'Here are some leaflets for you. Support groups. This one's quite local. Perhaps, when you're ready, you might benefit from talking to others who have shared your experience, people who will understand what you have just gone through.'

She removed her glasses and shoved them up so they rested behind her fringe.

'Listen,' she said. 'People say some ridiculous things when you've had a miscarriage, things that you may see as insensitive, offensive, hurtful. The best way to deal with it is to let it go over your head. They think they're trying to help. Don't let it get to you.'

I nodded, incapable of speech.

'And you're crying now, not keeping it all in. It might not feel like it, but it's a healthy reaction.'

My saddened and bowed husband walked in then. He sat with me, kissed me and held my hand.

'Well, I'd better leave you both now,' the social worker said. 'Here's my department number if you need to talk to me again. About anything.'

She touched my husband on the shoulder. 'Look after each other,' she said, but I felt she said it more to him than me. She looked at me a final time and I recognised something about her. Something shared.

It's happened to you too, hasn't it? I know it.

She left.

Perhaps she's never had a miscarriage. Perhaps she's just good at empathy. Good at her job.

It didn't take long before I received the first sledgehammer comment I had been warned to expect. I was explaining the story of my miscarriage to an acquaintance quite soon after it had happened. I told her what blighted ova were.

'Is that what they call a phantom pregnancy then?' she asked.

I felt like saying, 'What? Do you think I'm crazy? Do you think my body would pretend to be pregnant? Do you want to see my pregnancy test? I *have* kept my stinky stick with the two pink lines on it, you know. I can get it right now!'

But I remembered the words of the social worker back at the hospital and instead I said, 'No it's not like that. It's not like that at all.' I didn't bother explaining any further.

Six weeks later I went for a follow-up appointment at the hospital. I felt fine, but I thought I'd better front-up for the results of the pathology sample taken from the D and C. The doctor who saw me was young. She could have been fresh out of medical school.

'It says on your pathology report that there was no viable tissue.'

What was personal to me suddenly sounded so clinical, so cold. My 'loss wound' opened up again and I began to weep. There was nothing in my womb that was going to turn into a living baby—that's what 'no viable tissue' actually meant.

'Oh, don't worry,' she said waving a box of paper hankies towards me, 'you *will* be pregnant one day.'

'I *was* pregnant.'

'No, it says here, no viable tissue.'

Let it go over your head. Don't let it get to you.

I went on to have a further three miscarriages. And I have

Butterfly Nets   131

been on the receiving end of a lot of regrettable comments, just as the social worker said I would.

Others who have also experienced miscarriages said things like, 'I had a miscarriage but I was practical about it. Not meant to be is it? I just got on with life.' For a woman approaching the end of her reproductive days, it was extremely difficult to shrug off a miscarriage and get on with things. These kinds of 'ah, well' comments completely negated the emotions I felt at the time. I bonded with each of my pregnancies as soon as they began. As impractical and unrealistic as it was, each of my never-to-be babies had a name and it was always a wrench to leave them behind.

And then there were others who shared that they had also had a miscarriage, but theirs was somehow much worse. We are all women who have lost our babies, have mourned them, and will probably have a slight gnawing feeling of emptiness forever. Miscarriage isn't something to get competitive about when mutual support is needed.

As a former midwife it's difficult to say it, but there were two comments made by those in the medical and nursing professions that required me to call upon all my reserves of self-control when my nerves were raw with fresh grief.

Waiting to be wheeled into theatre after my fourth miscarriage, a junior anaesthetist was going through his checklist to see if there was any risk I might die on the table. When he'd finished he looked at me in a concerned way and said, 'I notice that you're looking very uptight, would you like a sedative to calm you down?'

I narrowed my eyes and said dangerously through gritted teeth: 'I-HAVE-JUST-HAD-A-MISCARRIAGE!'

He went away pretty soon after that and I hope he learned from me that some women going for a post-miscarriage D and C, particularly if they have suffered multiple miscarriages, can sometimes be a little on edge and extra sad and that it's really okay. It's not like I was running amok in the hospital corridors!

Next I had to deal with the comment of a perioperative nurse. I arrived at the theatre reception area on a trolley following my encounter with the anaesthetist. The nurse checked me in and helped the hospital porter wheel me to a bay to wait my turn. After telling me how sorry she was, she launched into a story about how she got pregnant at forty-five and had a miscarriage. 'I don't know how I would have coped anyway at that age,' she said. 'It's far too old to have a baby. You might be upset now, but believe me it's for the best.' She patted my shoulder.

Not only was I nowhere near forty-five (in fact I was a mere youngster of forty), but there was never a more inappropriate time to say it was *for the best*. I failed to comprehend how anybody could believe those words offered comfort. But I was cool, I was calm, I bore it well. I remembered the words of the social worker from three miscarriages ago and I just 'went with it' as she advised.

On the flipside, I have also met many people who have found just the right thing to say, and they were an enormous comfort to me. The most helpful people were those who simply said they were sorry, acknowledged my feelings and showed that they were fully present; those people who sat with me, who through the language of their bodies conveyed the message, *I am with you.*

The social worker—whose name I don't recall, but who is nevertheless etched in my mind—taught me how to be philosophical, taught me forbearance, taught me how to rise above outrage at others' want of wisdom and sense. These are some of the qualities required of a good parent.

Now the mother of two healthy, happy children, perfect in all (okay, most) ways, I have had plenty of opportunity to put the lessons I learned through my miscarriage experiences into practice. For this, especially, I would like to thank that nameless social worker very much.

Tracey Slater lives in Sydney with her husband, two kids and dog called Cosmo. A former nurse and midwife, she now assists with a primary school literacy program and is training to work as a teacher's aide. Tracey runs a writing group at the NSW Writers' Centre in Rozelle and is also a children's author.

Escaping from Good Friday
Heather Murray Tobias

I watched her load the surfboard into the car. It was hard to believe she was already in her mid-thirties: short tousled hair, lean brown body, her gender hidden by a loose T-shirt and baggy shorts. Laz rested his arm on my shoulder as I called out, 'Stay safe.' She waved and was gone.

Easter was always challenging. The traffic, the tourists, the way food disappeared from the supermarket shelves so rapidly, and there were the memories. No longer dwelt on or analysed but still there, hovering under the surface.

It was Good Friday. We picked up Mum, and I bundled myself into the back seat, smiling as my own precious passenger stirred inside my womb. The warm April sun beamed through the open windows of our VW, beetling its way up the Gully road. I shouted over the noise of the rear engine, enjoying the change of temperature and the heavy eucalyptus-laden air as we entered the forest.

There wasn't much leg room in the back seat and my old pelvic injury started a dull nag, increasing in intensity by the time we reach our driveway. Jedda, our kelpie-border collie cross, greeted us with great enthusiasm. Laz looked at me with a slight frown.

—You okay?

—Just my back, you know ... not able to stretch out. I'll be fine. Shshsh! Don't want Mum to fuss.

We made a salad of fresh greens and tomatoes from our garden, and hard-boiled eggs from our chooks. Mum and Laz were chatting but I couldn't find enthusiasm for food or conversation and made some excuse about having a late lunch. I rarely took painkillers, believing in mind over matter, but occasionally my back would insist and this was one of those moments.

I played some records, laughed at the dog and cat's antics—their regular game that left a trail of screwed-up mats and bed covers. The pain didn't subside. Doubts nibbled at a deep-buried memory. It couldn't be happening again. I had warned my doctor about my previous miscarriage but he had brushed my concerns aside.

—It's common to miscarry with your first, he said.

—Even at twenty-two weeks? And what about my family history?

—I'll keep an eye on you.

But had he? When I went to him recently reporting a show

of old blood he had checked the cervix and said everything was intact. Had he missed something?

The pain intensified again. I wanted to pass urine but couldn't. Was it something to do with my bladder?

And then I felt a gush of fluid.

Now I panicked. The hospital was about fifteen miles away through an autumn fog along winding forest roads. I remembered the last miscarriage all those years ago—a Singer sports car and how difficult it was to get out of it at the hospital.

Laz rang a neighbour, and within minutes I was in their Chev, speeding down the mountain. The pains increased in frequency and I lost my baby minutes after arrival. I heard the midwives whispering about the removal of the 'remains'. There was shock; a surreal detachment as I lay in a darkened room wrapped warmly.

A gynaecologist took over. He spoke kindly, preparing me mentally for a curette the next day and assuring me I could do this again with a positive outcome.

—I think I'll stick to my four-legged babies from now on if you don't mind.

He may have been shocked but I didn't care. I had been trying to conceive for eight years and I was now thirty-six. Who was this strange man, a latecomer on the scene, to tell me that I could bring a child into the world successfully. This man who didn't know the details of that first miscarriage seventeen years ago, of both grandmothers' miscarriages or early-term births, of my aunt's and my first cousin's hormonal irregularities that matched my own.

When they let Laz in we cried, together, empty of words.

The specialist had told him there was a procedure that could help me carry full-term. I didn't want to know. They weren't there that first time—none of them. It was of an earlier marriage, one I wanted to forget, and now I was drowning in the irony. Exactly seventeen years ago on the same day, on Good Friday, I lost my first son.

Back then, a friend drove us across the suburbs to the Women's Hospital. In the early hours of Good Friday the pains stopped. And I thought everything would be okay, but it wasn't. I was poked and prodded, my blood pressure and temperature were taken regularly, the baby's heartbeat monitored. Then it stopped.

Memories of trauma are frequently muddled or exquisitely clear. Mine is a mixture of both. I sharply recall the midwife's reluctance to tell me the baby's gender.

—Why won't you tell me?

—Because if you never have another child of that gender you may always grieve for the one you lost.

Why I would grieve for a gender, rather than a child, made no sense to me. I insisted on knowing.

—It was a little boy, came the gentle reply.

She shook her head. I was young there was lots of time to try again. There was nothing more to say.

I was in hospital for more than a week. I shared a ward with seven other women, all with their babes nuzzling and keening. The smell of newborns and milk—my own included—should have made me weep. Yet I didn't. Life took on a dream-like quality, the type of dream where you run away but go nowhere. Days dragged. This was 1956. Television was still seven months away and my love of books had deserted me.

Missionaries of various faiths moved through the ward, offering platitudes and I, reared a Methodist, found solace only in the words of a Catholic priest. He came twice and stayed, my denomination irrelevant. He chose not to discriminate, speaking quietly, not preaching, not sanctimonious—caring about me.

My mother came every day. My husband only twice. The hospital was too far for my car-less grandmother and aunt. My predicament at eighteen was not shared with my younger cousins or my brother. This is how it was, pregnancy was a confinement. Women enveloped themselves in flowing garments that concealed their 'condition', appearing in public only for the essentials of life—to attend medical appointments and maybe church.

When I was discharged the doctor told my husband that I may not be able to have any more children. He didn't speak to me, only to a man who was probably too drunk to understand the precise message.

I was dazed, floating in and out of disbelief. Existing in an empty, silent bubble. My physical body came into contact with those around me. I heard myself speak meaningless words, ate without tasting, touched and was touched without feeling. I watched life from a distant place. And no one knew.

Two weeks later the bleeding became a severe haemorrhage—the hospital had missed a piece of placenta.

Our toilet was outside and no one missed me. They were listening to *The Goon Show*, a weekly ritual.

The local doctor would not come and I was taken in the back of that Singer sports car to Emergency. I think I died in the car. I was experiencing a journey through darkness where an undefined presence helped me pass into bright light.

In the car, my mother was slapping my face, shaking me. The voice of the driver swearing and saying, Where are the bloody cops when you need them.

I remember not wanting to wake up, remember hearing my mother's muffled voice in the distance. I briefly regained consciousness at the hospital when our friend half-dragged half-lifted me out of his car and carried me into Emergency.

The mysterious bright light that was leading me through ethereal images faded and hands barred my way. There was a flurry of staff calling my name, running beside the trolley, injecting me.

Wrapped in blankets packed with hot water bottles I spent the night with a young nurse beside me, monitoring my blood pressure and temperature every half hour.

And then I was alert, everything sharply in focus. A soft night-light cast shadows along the walls of the balcony which housed many beds. The ward was filled with the sounds of the traffic below, the crisp whispers of starched bed linen, and the other patients— all women who had miscarried or were too ill to return home. But the miasma that had surrounded me since Good Friday lifted.

The experience that bought me so close to death also gave me back my life. My marriage had removed me from the tight-knit family circle that was formed by twins, my mother and aunt. There was no approval for my husband. Even his own parents disapproved of the way he treated me. The relationship could not, did not, last.

I freed myself and eventually secured a travel industry job that was exciting and glamorous. I joined an amateur theatre company. For the next nine years all thoughts of motherhood were deeply buried as I pursued every moment, grabbing life with both hands, with all the energy I could muster.

The close touch of death deepened my understanding of what was truly important, the things that couldn't be bought. It reignited my childhood interest in the simple creatures who shared our need for a healthy, natural environment and the realisation that all negative experience has a positive aspect.

Then I met a Hungarian refugee who, born in the same year, shared a similar family structure, even though our childhoods had been separated by a hemisphere, a war and cultural differences. We shared an interest in self-sufficiency, freedom and equality.

We worked hard, focused on owning our own home. That achieved I left work, deciding to pursue a long-neglected interest in art, unaware that I was pregnant. But now he was taking me home from hospital, empty again and silent, sadness closing a palpable wall around me.

Menstruation did not start again after my second miscarriage. I was unconcerned. I had lived with erratic periods since I was ten years old—nothing for months and then periods every two weeks, and then nothing for a long time again.

My days were filled with gardening, painting, and looking after pets and chooks. Then in July, my beloved dog Jedda was killed on our newly-made road. It was too soon, too painful. The emptiness returned.

But I was not empty. Unrecognised, my daughter had started her long struggle for survival. Forty-eight days of her gestation, of my 'confinement', were spent in hospital, and at the end she was laid in the arms of her awestruck mother, on a hot March day, too early for Easter.

Today, a surfboard protruded from the car window, the wheels left behind a trail of dust, carrying her to a rendezvous with bliss—a wild ride on a wave.

Heather Murray Tobias completed BA majors in Literary Studies and History of Art and Architecture at Deakin University. She was the coordinator for Ibis Writers and the concept creator of its inaugural writing festival in Cowes. Her poems, short stories and articles have been published in a number of anthologies and journals, and her debut collection of poetry, A Feather in My Hair, *was published earlier this year by Thoth's Quill.*

Unexpected

Clare McHugh

Our daughter Julia cuts the pomegranate bought at the Bastille Markets. Such colour and delight is barely believable in the dim Paris winter. Around the small table set against the apartment's wall, the three of us tuck in. Soon red seeds spurt everywhere. The white lampshade, white curtain and wall are spattered. Every time her father digs in with his spoon to scoop crunchy seeds—'They taste like life itself,' he says—more red juice bursts in all directions. Hardly pausing to talk, we giggle, scrape and slurp. Julia suggests pomegranate seeds should always be eaten in the bath, on Valentine's Day, with the beloved. Her father thinks the beach would be perfect. We grunt agreement while chasing down each last seed. Easy to see how just a few of these seeds kept wilful Persephone in the underworld.

Being with Julia again, away from the rest of life, just the three of us, sends me back to an earlier time, before the baby that disappeared. When it was just Andrew, Julia and me. For now though we're escaping one long winter and a year of near-death, by entering a new year and a second winter. We have come to see our daughter's student habitat and, as an afterthought, mark the calendar clicking over twenty-five years of married life. Paris was to be the antiveneme to an unexpected year spent with doctors and rehab nurses, hovering in waiting rooms, poring over angiograms.

Mostly we have come to erase the memory of her father's frailty and the uncertainty that hung in the air as Julia left Australia all those months ago. But Paris had unexpected plans.

He seems so fit. Even in the cold of that afternoon as we laugh at blood-like spatterings on rented walls, last year's surgery is just a slim pink scar the length of his torso.

Then Andrew is unexpectedly laid low once more. His retreat to bed gives an unexpected pause for turning over a lifetime of medical experiences that once seemed like isolated disasters but are now simply part of the bibliography. Reference points to consult during other events.

The baby that never arrived twenty years ago no longer troubles me as it did. There are plenty of recent troubles and with two, nearly three, adult children and a husband who didn't die, plenty to be grateful for. It seems cheap or somehow dishonourable to chase a small long-ago grief that has settled into the silt; to deliberately disinter.

Over time the baby, the sadness of those months, have been like a room that gradually falls out of use in a house of busy rooms. Life has surged on around it. The room remains, full of trinkets and familiar furnishings that can cause a gasp of surprise on revisiting, but with no reason to linger there it receives no more than a cursory glance from time to time. Other rooms with more pressing tasks call for attention. From a family of five we have dwindled in recent months to a solitary schoolboy eyeing the calendar and a 'gap year'.

When Andrew's recovery seems to stall, our daughter calls the emergency doctor. I listen and watch, like the toddler this trip has made me, as Julia's French persona takes over. Familiar and unfamiliar words rear up. I understand their drift but not the detail.

Within an hour an elegant and efficient young woman arrives. She looks concerned when I urge *asthmatique, cardiac*. Julia sighs and converts my pantomime to words. What is the French for *pleural effusion*? The doctor nods and frowns.

We pass the twenty-five-year milestone with Andrew alone and feverish in the apartment and me alone in cafés. He is uninterested in most things but loves our daughter's conversation; snippets about her study or morsels read to him from the Web.

Last year we listened as surgeons—humane, confident, assured—dangled procedures, risks, their supreme skills in front of us. A one in one hundred chance of dying this way; a two in one hundred chance of dying another way. I listened and calculated. The risks seemed high but of course, they assure cheerfully, you'll definitely die if we do nothing. Won't we all.

He spent months after surgery, willing and working his way back to life. But will is sometimes not enough. Twenty years ago I willed it to be all right. Went to bed. Lay still. Felt hope and fear in equal parts. A doctor's words and a scan the next day confirmed what we had begun to know. With regrets expressed and a referral for surgery, we were sent home to wait for the next available date. Later at home that night in painful spasms, as if the doctor's strange words had broken a fifteen-week spell, broken whatever force was holding it all together, the pregnancy ended.

Fragments of that endless night remain, of things slipping away, of feeling sad and hopeless at not being able to stop it happening. I was young, healthy and had carried one baby to term, but willing and hoping, health and youth were not enough.

On a freezing late autumn day twenty years ago, I clenched and unclenched my fists as instructed, while a flustered intern tried to insert an intravenous drip and told me I had bad veins. Nothing worked as intended. A sense of failing descended. Well-meaning medical staff underlined it several times.

Didn't you realise that the pregnancy had not progressed for some weeks?

Didn't you feel a difference?

Did you sense a drop in the hormone levels?

A sudden surge of energy?

Harsh words like marbles in my mouth. *Cytoblast. Not a viable gestation. A collection of cells.* The doctor kept circling down stairways of meaning away from his screens and scans towards us. We looked at him, waiting for meaning although it had already arrived.

'It was not really a human form.' The final blow. As if we'd made it up. Our bodies had made up something but not what was expected.

It felt like losing love. Loving someone, waiting for them, only to find that they weren't going to show. Feeling desolate and foolish in the expectation.

Life comes down to this frail boat that we sail in. The surgeons and nurses, efficient and watchful, do so much. It seems they can hold back the sea for our safe crossing but we must first set sail. For heart surgery, for asthma, for pneumonia, whether French or Australian, they know what is to be done and what will heal. Yet when that baby was disappearing, everyone could only stand back and murmur awkward regrets. The ultrasound technician muttered about getting the doctor and left the room. After a year in the hands of masterful and persistent health professionals I am struck by their acceptance of miscarriage, their resignation at the mystery of life begun in darkness, hidden.

Whole hospitals of skilled people can incubate, vent, insert grafts and pump lungs but each of us has to take hold of life first. Some lose their grip and fall away early, some before they can begin ...

The fumbling words of others and my reactions come back; the deep grief that settled and felt as if it would never go away.

There will be other babies.

Yes, but not this one.

My friend has been diagnosed with cancer. She was hoping for a new kitchen this year, instead she'll have a new breast. My husband lies seriously ill. Has anyone ever offered the consolation that there will be other breasts, other friends, other husbands?

Rallying well-intended words are offered to diminish invisible losses. A baby conceived in darkness. A young heart, broken in ways that adults know will never be quite the same, is told, *There are plenty of fish in the sea*. But what they want is the one that is swimming away, out of reach and out of love. How often I have spoken similar clumsy words, tried to adjust, reframe, instead of listen.

Its nature's way of cleaning up her mistakes.

Yes. That fact strikes home. *More difficult things could happen.*

One in four pregnancies ends in miscarriage a scientist friend told me. His short Yorkshire sentences succeeded where others failed: consoling by trying not to. The figure could be as high as one in two, he said. This made me see everyone differently. Comfort in cold data. How many women there were out there who had been through this. It cast different light on sad, distracted faces at bus stops, carrying shopping, ignoring or rebuking a child.

The slight pause between our first and second daughters caused comment over the years. Perhaps it was the trend then to cram the baby years together. Three under four years and back to work when school began. Whatever the reason, that little gap—like a gap between teeth that is visible but not bad enough for braces—stayed as a reminder. A little bump in the road to children like an unmarked mound in a cemetery.

Then a child arrived. A child that could not have existed if the lost one had. That is the slow truth although it takes a long time to take seed. There is no use fighting losses, not even fighting to understand them. Only acceptance and gratitude for the rest.

I meet our daughter after class or work and follow her to a new particular place for a glass of wine or rare tea. We make the best of the time with each other. We arrange medical appointments for Andrew. She consults French colleagues but we do not talk much about what if. We try not to think too far ahead, about the long plane trip home and how Andrew will make it.

On one of those days I stand waiting for Julia outside her university residence. The day is bleak and yet across the narrow austerity of the street, from behind a single heavy door comes the sound of children laughing and chattering. It is play time across the road at the *ecole maternelle*.

A darkly marble plaque with a flag and a bouquet high on the wall of the school draws my eye. For a moment I labour until the French expressions yield. In memory of the children rounded up between 1942 and 1944 because they were born Jewish. Innocent victims of the Nazi barbarism with the active complicity of the Vichy French government.

Taken from this school, barely visible behind its blank stone façade. Their lives swept away before they were begun.

In the days that follow the plaque weighs on me and I notice many more. In a park across the river from Notre Dame a transparent obelisk lists the names of children too young to attend school, also taken and exterminated in the death camps. Irene and Rosette, four years and one year, are sisters. Others aged five, three, four also taken.

Resisting, acceptance and gratitude take a new turn. Who is to say what can be wished for; what can be hung onto by force of will? This little tossed about boat we ride in is fragile, designed to fail one day, naturally. That is not disaster. That is design. Malice, madness and cruelty, and the failure to see it—that is disaster.

Outside that school as I wait for my own clever daughter to skip down the stairs and smile at me, it's not only the frigid air that pricks my eyes. I breathe in a deep lungful; grateful for now, for near misses and far misses, knowing that kind-faced doctors may one day again stand over me and shrug off their helplessness.

'Sorry I've kept you,' she says planting a big kiss on my cheek and we link arms and head off along the river.

In the days that follow the three of us wrestle with the decision to return but finally choose to risk a long flight rather than wait for Andrew to remake himself yet again: something we are not sure will happen soon. At home the school term is beginning for our son. Our second daughter—that vivacious child that could not exist if the lost baby did—has announced a move to Melbourne. There is another room to pack up, another person on their way. The coordinates on our map stretch further.

Clare McHugh is a professional writer, editor and a consultant on family and children's issues. She works for a commercial publisher and her nonfiction covers online and print articles—mostly on families, relationships and social policy—as well as two short fiction pieces.

The Long Wait

Deb Nurton

I like a story with a happy ending.

In fact, this is so important to me that if I am watching a movie or reading a book and I sense that everything is not going to turn out okay, I skip to the end scene or page to make sure there are no surprises. Only then do I go back and finish the rest of the story, and so it's for the best that I tell you we now have two beautiful boys.

Ah, but those words. They come back to me through time: *It's for the best*. Those words have not always had such a simple fluency from my tongue. Those four little words haunted me back then, in the dark times.

So many people. So many well-meaning, good-intentioned people. 'It's for the best,' they told me over and over again. It was for the best that my little baby, my son or daughter, had for no apparent reason stopped developing at one day past the twelve-week mark, just when we thought we were 'in the clear'. Just like that. My baby had died, yet somehow I was to be comforted by the fact that it must have been malformed—some monstrous thing that could not, should not, be allowed to survive.

Why? I wanted to scream. Why was it for the best? Why did it have to be *my* baby, the one I had wanted for so long. There were, of course, no answers. I sat—devastated, dazed, delirious in the soft July afternoon sunlight—trying to come to terms with the news that there had been no heartbeat and so there was no hope.

Please remember, at this point, the happy ending.

At that time, I had been waiting for a baby for a very long time. A string of disastrous relationships behind me, at last I had found union with a truly lovely man. The trouble was that all those disastrous relationships had used up most of my child-bearing years, and now I had to get a wiggle on if I was to make a lucky catch from my ever-dwindling egg supply. I was teetering towards thirty-eight when the joyous moment of a blue line on a pregnancy test propelled me into panic about becoming a mother. Was I up to the task? Could I manage what lay before me? Was I ready?

The answers, unfortunately, were no, no and no.

I had waited so long to be pregnant, and now it seemed I was being asked to wait even longer. I wanted it out, as soon as possible, this ruined foetus, so I could go back to the drawing board and do it all again. Quickly, please.

Steely-eyed, I ventured yet again into the murky sea of sex-for-a-baby, my strength and confidence now more than a little diminished. But where we had struck it lucky after only three months of trying the first time, now the shock appearance of my monthlies went on and on and on interminably. To make the whole thing more difficult for us, my husband's oldest sister had been a month behind us in her due date for her baby, and her pregnancy carried on, a reminder of what we were missing out on. Then, out of the blue, my husband's other sister got pregnant by accident. So there they were at every family event, getting bigger and rounder and discussing babies in front of me. Understandable, of course, from their point of view, as they were excited about having their first children and my mother-in-law her first grandchildren. But their good fortune only emphasised our loss—our baby should not only have been among these babes-in-waiting, it should have been the first born, the oldest of them all.

Christmas rolled around and I decided I couldn't bear to be at a family gathering, on Christmas Day of all days, as the only one without a baby in her womb. I stayed home. My husband went. I found the peace and solitude soothing, although not the reason why I was home alone.

Remember, please, the happy ending.

Both of the new babies arrived. The anniversary of our miscarriage came and went. And still there was no pregnancy for us.

Now desperately clinging to my thirties, I went to visit a woman who thought she could help me. Not a doctor or any kind of health professional. Not even a naturopath. No, this little pixie of a woman steered me, over the next two months, through the agony of the emotional blocks she said were preventing me from achieving a pregnancy. She balanced my chakras and my hara and massaged my body to within an inch of its strength.

'What's a chakra?' my husband asked me. 'I have no idea,' I told him, 'but I am suspending my disbelief because it feels right to do this.'

Not long after, the fog seemed to clear and I became surprisingly more lucid in my thinking—enough to decide to change our focus. My obstetrician was very kind, but he continued to tell us I was the 'problem' and never investigated my husband's side of things. My husband offered again and again to have a sperm test, just to be sure of everything, but the obstetrician kept saying no.

In the end, we decided to take matters into our own hands and I rang the Reproductive Medicine Clinic at our local hospital. They were more than happy to do simple tests—on both of us. It turned out I was ovulating fine, even for my age, but my husband had a higher than usual abnormal sperm count. What did this mean for us? Was it dire news? It didn't matter because we felt we were suddenly on the road to somewhere.

That road was a new way forward. The clinic referred us to one of their specialists, an intelligent, caring, no-nonsense obstetrician who felt 'right' to us, a good fit, and we began to see a way through, although there was no good news.

Remember, after all, there is a happy ending.

He told us we probably had no chance of conceiving

naturally because of my age—I had just turned thirty-nine—and because of the results of the sperm test. He kindly recommended IVF—the kind where the embryo is fertilised outside the womb and then implanted—and we were given a swathe of information about it.

Funnily enough, we were not devastated by this news. Armed with information and choice, we decided not to pursue IVF. By this stage we were flying into unknown territory, being led only by our intuition and with little information in our favour. But we now set about doing whatever we thought was reasonable, even though there was not a lick of scientific evidence to back us up. My husband started wearing boxers. I continued to see my pixie woman. I lay in bed after sex, just to make sure the sperm had its chance to swim in the right direction without gravity acting against it.

Bingo! Within a few weeks we were pregnant.

Unfortunately, that one didn't even last as long as the first, and I was back in hospital again after seven weeks of pregnancy. This time, the obstetrician explained there was no foetal pole, which meant that a baby wasn't forming, just the amniotic sac and the placenta. But whereas with the first miscarriage I had been distraught, this time, although sad, I felt encouraged. I had a feeling we were on the right track. So did the obstetrician. 'Well, you've done it twice. Go home and see what you can do.' Armed again with new information about the best days for conception, we set about the task.

I had been studying through this entire period and, oddly enough, both miscarriages commenced with bleeding on the afternoon that I sat my final exam for each semester. So with degree in hand but no baby in arms, I decided to take a year off from everything. I would not continue on to Honours or look for work and we would leave a space for a baby to enter our lives.

In May of the following year, on a just-for-the-hell-of-it-let's-not-worry-about-the-whole-baby-thing-this-month wedding anniversary, we made love—and a baby.

Yes, we were scared throughout the entire pregnancy. Yes, the scans were so terrifying I nearly fainted. But we managed to hold it together for the full nine months and, eventually, at the age of forty, I became a first-time mother. I could write the most joyous of all words to describe our feelings on the birth of our son and still not come close to the exultation we experienced.

Then almost four years later, just as I turned forty-four, we found out we were again pregnant and another son was born the next year. This time he was a Father's Day conception!

In hindsight, if they were to come, I was glad the miscarriages happened before we had any children. I didn't think this at the time, of course. But I must admit, they did clear up any ideas I had about not being ready for motherhood. I was so ready by the time my eldest was born that I found the way clearer. And with time I came to be grateful for the gift that those two miscarriages gave me. They gave me time to pause and reflect that having a family was not a right but a privilege. Somehow, our struggle made the fruits all the sweeter.

So our two boys are precious—two special occasion conceptions, two gifts of love—and we feel very fortunate to have them in our lives. On days when motherhood has me rattled, cross, tired and grumpy, I stop for a moment and think what it would be like if we didn't have them—and the silence is deafening. They are well loved, well appreciated, and well worth the wait.

So, here at last, as promised, is the happy ending. Well, kind of. Because really birth is not an ending, but a beginning.

Deb Nurton holds degrees in teaching and psychology. She writes in a variety of forms about love, learning, parenting, childhood, and nature. Deb believes her greatest achievements are marrying her husband, raising two magnificent boys and reducing her family's carbon footprint.

Information and resources

Support organisations

Bonnie Babes Foundation
www.bonniebabes.org.au
Phone 1300 266 643 (24-hour helpline)
A non-profit charity which raises funds for medical research into pregnancy loss and complications, education for health professionals and support and counselling.

SANDS Australia
www.sands.org.au/
Phone 1300 072 637 (to talk to another bereaved parent)
Miscarriage, stillbirth and neonatal death support.

SIDS and Kids
www.sidsandkids.org
Phone 1300 308 307 (for 24-hour bereavement support and information)
SIDS and Kids provides support, information and research into saving the lives of babies and children during pregnancy, birth infancy and childhood.

Teddy Love Club
www.teddyloveclub.org.au
Phone 1800 824 240 (free call bereavement support 9am–6pm)
An Australia-wide support program for families who lose their baby during pregnancy or after birth. It runs a donate-a-bear program for bereaved parents.

Websites

Babyloss
www.babyloss.com
A UK-based site providing information and support for pregnancy and infant loss.

Bugaboo Jewelry
http://kristi-bugaboojewelry.blogspot.com/
Kristi Sagrillo makes contemporary memorial jewellery for families who, like hers, have lost a child.

Charing Cross Hospital
www.hmole-chorio.org.uk
Charing Cross Hospital in the UK is the leading specialist centre in molar pregnancies. Its website provides a reliable source of information on the disease and its treatment.

Essential Baby
www.essentialbaby.com.au
Essential Baby has a section for miscarriage and pregnancy loss and a forum to support women.

Faces of Loss, Faces of Hope
http://facesofloss.com/
A 'baby loss club' where people can read the stories, and see the faces of those who have experienced miscarriage, stillbirth and infant loss.

Facts About Miscarriage
http://pregnancyloss.info/
A site that provides 'information, healing and hope'. It houses a virtual memorial garden where parents can leave notes to their babies.

Glow in the woods
www.glowinthewoods.com
Support for parents who have lost a baby at any stage that includes discussion boards.

Infertility Network UK
www.infertilitynetworkuk.com/
The UK's leading infertility support network, offering information and support to anyone affected by fertility problems.

Molarpregnancy.co.uk
www.molarpregnancy.co.uk/info.html
A molar pregnancy support site that includes a forum.

Pregnancy and Infant Loss Remembrance Day
www.october15th.com
The official site of the international remembrance Day (October 15) which provides information and support.

Recurrent Miscarriages Information Center
www.recurrentmiscarriages.com
Information on miscarriage by Krissi Danielsson, author of *After Miscarriage*.

To Write Their Names in the Sand
www.namesinthesand.blogspot.com
A memorial website featuring photographs of the names of lost babies written in the sand at sunset.

Unspoken Grief
http://unspokengrief.com/
Created by Devan McGuinness, who experienced ten miscarriages, this site offers a place to 'share, talk, support and learn about the impact of miscarriage, stillbirth and neonatal loss'.

Blogs

Babyfruit: The (Mis)adventures of Mommyhood
http://babyfruit.typepad.com/baby
Aliza Risdahl's blog is about 'miscarriage blogging, miscarriage advice, celebrity miscarriage and other miscarrying obsessions. Throw in pregnancy, post partum depression, and now juggling life as a forty-something mom of a four-year-old'.

Miscarriage One Two Many
www.miscarriageonetwomany.blogspot.com/
Ashley Kingsley's blog is 'for the countless silent sufferers who have lost babies through miscarriage'.

Miscarriage, Stillbirth, and Infant Loss Directory
http://babylossdirectory.blogspot.com/
The blog is maintained by volunteers to act like a telephone book for blogs dealing with the loss of a baby.

Tuesday's Hope
www.tuesdayshope.blogspot.com
A blog about one woman's personal journey of miscarriage.

Whispered Support
www.whisperedsupport.blogspot.com
A blog providing practical and helpful information 'to guide you through the days surrounding the death of your precious baby'.

CPSIA information can be obtained at www.ICGtesting.com
Printed in the USA
LVOW04s2240010415

432911LV00024B/353/P